THE MEDEDITS GUIDE TO

THE MEDICAL SCHOOL INTERVIEW

MMI AND TRADITIONAL: EVERYTHING YOU NEED TO KNOW

JESSICA FREEDMAN, M.D.

CHAIR AND FOUNDER OF MEDEDITS MEDICAL ADMISSIONS

Some of the anecdotes I have used in this book are based on my actual experiences, but applicants' identities have been concealed. Some of this material, including the sample interview, is completely fictitious. Remember that plagiarism is illegal so do not regurgitate any of the information provided in this book for your actual interview or in your application materials. Authenticity is essential for your success so plagiarizing, even if you aren't "caught," will jeopardize your chances of admission. The information in this book does not guarantee that you will be accepted to medical school.

ABOUT THE AUTHOR

Jessica Freedman, MD is a former associate residency director and faculty member at the Icahn Mount Sinai School of Medicine in New York City. A top rated faculty member at Mount Sinai, she served on the medical school admissions committee and was involved in medical education and curriculum design at the graduate and undergraduate levels. She is also a published author and has served on national committees related to medical education. Dr. Freedman is president and founder of MedEdits Medical Admissions, the nation's top private advising company for applicants to medical school, residency and fellowship. MedEdits has helped hundreds of successful medical school applicants gain admission to medical school. Dr. Freedman is an emergency physician and lives in New York.

HOW CAN MEDEDITS HELP YOU?

1. We are constantly updating our website and offering additional information that is useful for premeds, medical students, and residents. Visit our website often (mededits. com) and sign up for our newsletter.
2. Read Dr. Freedman's books, The MedEdits Guide to

Medical School Admissions and How to Be an All-Star Residency Match Applicant.

3. Work with MedEdits Medical Admissions to receive personalized help on every step of the medical school admissions process.

WHAT DISTINGUISHES MEDEDITS?

1. All of our faculty members have served on medical school admissions committees for a MINIMUM of five years at the faculty level. We never hire recent medical school graduates, physicians with distant or minimal medical school admissions experience.

2. We stay up to date with trends in medical school admissions by attending national meetings, reading the academic medicine literature, and collaborating with our colleagues.

3. MedEdits faculty are well versed in all types of medical school interviews.

TABLE OF CONTENTS

ACRONYMS

This book uses many acronyms, including the following:

AACOMAS®: American Association of Colleges of Osteopathic Medicine Application Service

AAMC: Association of American Medical Colleges

AMCAS®: American Medical College Application Service

AO: All other (refers to GPA)

BCPM: Biology, chemistry, physics, math (refers to GPA)

CASPer: Computer-Based Assessment for Sampling Personal Characteristics

COMLEX®: Comprehensive Osteopathic Medical Licensing Exam

CV: Curriculum Vitae

DO: Doctor of Osteopathy

FAFSA®: Free Application for Federal Student Aid

FAP: Fee Assistance Program

GPA: Grade point average

MCAT®: Medical College Admission Test

MD: Doctor of Medicine

MMI: Multiple Mini Interview

MPH: Master of Public Health

NRMP®: National Residency Matching Program

PBL: Problem based learning

PhD: Doctor of Philosophy

TMDSAS®: Texas Medical & Dental Application Service

USMLE®: United States Medical Licensing Exam

INTRODUCTION

My goal in writing this new edition the The Medical School Interview is to offer medical school applicants a comprehensive guide that would provide everything you need to know while not overwhelming the reader. The vast majority of medical school applicants will have two types of interviews during the admission process: the traditional medical school interview and the multiple mini interview (MMI). The thought of preparing for medical school interviews can be daunting for applicants and this guide will help to prepare you so you know what to expect and feel confident and eager for your medical school interviews.

I started my "interview career" as an interviewee myself when I was a premedical student and then again as a residency applicant, but I learned most about this process during the 10 years I spent in the interviewer's seat and as an interview coach and mentor to medical school applicants through MedEdits Medical Admissions. Like most physicians, I had no formal training or experience when I started interviewing candidates. During my years of selecting candidates, I learned what qualities applicants must have to interview well. More important, however, I learned what goes on behind the scenes after interview day and how a candidate's success is affected by the interviewer's skills and experience. Indeed, I gained an understanding of how both experienced and inexperienced interviewers evaluate applicants and what applicants can do to influence these differences to their advantage. After working with applicants who are preparing for interviews with www.MedEdits. com, I also know what mistakes interviewees commonly make, what insecurities applicants have and which applicants do well in the interview setting. Our experience coaching thousands of successful medical school applicants also gives insight about what, and how much, students need to prepare to do well in the process. There is a fine line between under preparation and over preparation and often the key is knowing when you are "ready" which is not easy for the majority of premedical students.

These experiences, from both the "outside" and the "inside," allow me to provide a unique perspective to medical school applicants who are preparing for interviews. Thus, this book, based on my inside understanding of the medical admissions process and my work privately advising students, is a must-read for both interviewees and interviewers alike. It covers everything you need to know, beginning with what you should do to prepare for interview day, what to expect on The Day, and the nitty gritty of how to behave during and after the interview. By having a full understanding of the medical school admissions process, knowing what goes on behind the scenes before and after your interview, who will be interviewing you, what the interviewer is looking for and what you can do to influence how your interview will progress, you will be better prepared to do well and present yourself in the best light.

A NOTE FOR THE INTERVIEWER

I encourage medical school interviewers to read this book to gain some insight into how to make thorough, accurate, and complete assessments of medical school applicants when you interview them. I find that many medical student interviewers and first time attending interviewers are often as nervous as the applicants! Based on my own experience in academic medicine, I know that we typically receive no training on how to interview applicants. In fact, I sometimes found myself teaching my senior attendings about how to review an application and interview an applicant to make sure all important information was obtained and to rule out any red flags.

There are always applicants who have "slipped through the cracks" when the admission committee failed to notice a significant piece of their history. These applicants may have difficulty in medical school or residency or as attendings, and it is therefore the interviewer's responsibility to make sure such individuals are identified. Failure to do so not only compromises a seat in a medical school or residency class when a student cannot complete a portion of his or her education but may also negatively affect patient care. I work primarily with applicants, but I have also helped friends and colleagues to refine and improve their interviewing and application reviewing skills.

PART 1:

INTERVIEW BASICS

CHAPTER 1

WHO GETS INVITED FOR AN INTERVIEW?

The first step of the medical school admissions process is to compose a written application and to send, along with those documents, transcripts and letters of reference. There are three primary application systems:

1. AMCAS - The American Medical School College Application Service
    -This application is used to apply to all allopathic medical school in the United States except Texas medical schools, excluding Baylor
2. AACOMAS – Association of Colleges of Osteopathic Medicine Application Service.
    -This application system is used to apply to all osteopathic medical schools in the United States except Texas.
3. TMDSAS - Texas Medical and Dental Schools Application Service
    -This system is used to apply to all medical schools in Texas except Baylor.

Your written application, which is reviewed to determine if you should be invited for an interview, consists of:

1. Biographic information
2. List of courses and grades
3. List of activities and accomplishments and descriptions of each
4. Personal statement
5. Explanations for other circumstances such as a misdemeanor or underserved status
6. Transcripts
7. Letters of Recommendation

A wide range of people screen medical school applications and decide who should be invited for an interview, including current medical students, attending physicians, medical school administrators and basic scientists. Some schools and programs have minimum cutoffs for grades and standardized test scores, and the application of anyone who does not reach these levels does not even make it to the screening process. Some schools assign "points" for everything: extracurricular activities, medical college admissions test (MCAT) scores, and letters of recommendation; you are invited for an interview only when your score meets a minimum number. More often, whatever the grading system, a great deal of subjectivity goes into the decision to invite an applicant for an interview. Frequently, the screener's personal interests and outlook play a part in the review of your application--especially if you are a "borderline" applicant. For example, if reviewer A always had to struggle with standardized tests yet managed to succeed while reviewer B always had board scores in the top fifth percentile, reviewer A is much more likely than reviewer B to screen in an application with lower-than-average board scores.

The person reading your application might have years of admissions experience or he or she could be a novice, such as a medical student or a junior faculty member. Both the level of experience of the screener and his own biases and preferences often determine whether or not you are granted an interview. Also, although the person reading your application might have hours to peruse through all of your materials, it is more likely that she is tired and rushed and has a large pile of applications to review. If your application follows one that is more stellar, yours may pale in comparison. On the other hand, if the pile contains mostly mediocre-to-poor applications, yours may stand out.

For all of these reasons, making your application as distinctive as possible increases the likelihood you will be invited for an interview. If the application bores the person reading it, you will likely end up in the rejection pile. But you must also understand that many applicants to medical school are highly qualified and that many steps in the selection process are out of your control. This is a hard truth to accept, and you can only hope that your application and letters of reference are appealing enough to trigger some medical school interview invitations. Each interview is a chance for acceptance, so it is essential to be prepared and know what to expect.

To increase your chances of getting interviews, I suggest reading my medical school admissions book, The MedEdits Guide to Medical School Admissions. This book outlines what you should do to improve your candidacy and your written application which is what will dictate your success in receiving the most medical school interview invitations.

There are many factors that determine who is invited to interviews at any specific medical school. Below are average metrics for medical school matriculants from all three application systems for 2017, the most recent data available when this book was written. These data do not change significantly from year to year.

Allopathic medical school matriculant averages (AMCAS):

MCAT®: 510.4 (CPBS: 127.6, CARS: 126.9, BBLS: 127.9, PSBB: 128.0)
GPA Science: 3.64
GPA Non-Science: 3.79
GPA Total: 3.71

Osteopathic medical school matriculant averages (AACOMAS):

MCAT®: 503.05 (CPBS: 125.68, CARS: 125.2, BBLS: 126, PSBB: 126.17)
GPA Science: 3.43
GPA Non-Science: 3.64
GPA Total: 3.53

Texas medical school matriculant averages (TMDSAS):

MCAT: 509.1 (CBPS: 127.3, CARS: 126.6, BBLS: 127.5, PSBB: 127.6)

GPA Science: 3.64
GPA Total: 3.75

When deciding where to apply, it is important to be honest with yourself. For which medical schools, and which types of medical schools, are you most competitive? If necessary, what can you do to make yourself a more competitive applicant?

Once you reach the interview stage of the medical school admission process, it means you have passed all "screenings" to get to that stage. It also means you possess the academic credentials required by the medical school. Congratulations! From that point on, your "interview performance" and how you are perceived on interview day will be the most critical factor in your success.

If you want to read more about what makes a great medical school applicant, read, The MedEdits Guide to Medical Admissions.

CHAPTER 2

WHAT ARE THE DIFFERENT TYPES OF INTERVIEWS?

You typically will know in advance what type of interview each school conducts, which should help to prepare you psychologically and literally. Below are the five major types of interviews.

TRADITIONAL INTERVIEWS

The majority of interviews are "traditional" one on one interviews. These interviews are most commonly a question and answer format and often transition into conversational interviews or discussions. Traditional interviews fall into one of three categories - open, closed, or partially closed file

1) TRADITIONAL OPEN FILE INTERVIEW

An open file interview is the most common type. In an open file interview, the interviewer has access to all of your information, including all written documents, letters of reference, and test scores. But just because an interview is open file does not mean that the interviewer has read all of your materials. Your interview is just one part of his day, and if the interviewer was awakened at 2 AM for an emergency, he probably has not had time to read through your file. Or, maybe your interviewer was teaching a class that ran late, and he had only five minutes to review your materials. You must prepare for an open file interview in the same way you would for a closed file interview (discussed below). Do not assume that your interviewer knows a thing about you. Also, do not be offended if your interviewer reads your file while you are speaking. This may be the first time he has glimpsed your personal statement, application, and letters of reference. Many students think it is best to abbreviate responses during an open file interview since the interviewer has access to all of your background information. However, this is not the correct approach. It is best to walk into an open file interview as if the interviewer knows nothing about you. First of all, as I have mentioned, the interviewer may have skimmed or read nothing of your application. Secondly, the interviewer wants to know that you, the interviewee, "match" what he or she has read in your application.

2) TRADITIONAL CLOSED FILE INTERVIEW

In this type of interview, the interviewer may have no or limited access to your materials. These interviews therefore offer an opportunity to control the interview and dictate what is discussed. Most closed file interviews follow some sort of pattern. The interviewer may either have a set list of questions he or she is supposed to ask you or the interviewer has her own style of how to conduct an interview and has set questions she likes to ask. Regardless of the type of interview, open or closed file, your approach to the interview should not differ.

3) TRADITIONAL PARTIALLY CLOSED FILE INTERVIEW

Partially closed file interviews typically mean that the interviewer has everything except your MCAT and GPA; however, this varies from school to school.

4) PANEL INTERVIEW

Applicants tend to find a panel interview more intimidating than any other type. Typically, the panel comprises three interviewers and one interviewee. In these types of interviews, all interviewees are asked the same questions. The reason for a panel interview is because it's an efficient way for several people to evaluate an applicant at the same time. How this interview proceeds depends in part on the dynamic and hierarchy of the interviewers. For example, a junior faculty member may be intimidated by a more senior faculty member and therefore may be more concerned with her own performance than with the interviewee's. It is important during these interviews not to psychoanalyze the group who is interviewing you but to stay focused on their questions and your own personal agenda of what you hope to convey.

5) GROUP INTERVIEW

These interviews typically involve several interviewers and interviewees. Their objective is to see how you manage pressure and how you respond to others. You should listen attentively to everyone's answers and be a team player. If someone gives an answer that you wanted to give, make a joke: "John just gave my answer and now I have nothing to say." Do not act as though the other interviewees are competitors. Listen respectfully to what they have to say, make eye contact and be interested in everyone. Though it is natural to compare yourself with other interviewees in the group, be aware that the other interviewees' answers may "sound better" than your own not because they actually are superior to your answers but because their stories are new to you.

6) MULTIPLE MINI INTERVIEWS

This type of interview was developed in Canada, and more and more medical schools in the United States use it. Students rotate through a variety of "stations," remaining at each for eight to 10 minutes to address a particular question, complete a task, or work with another student. For example, the interviewer may give you a scenario and ask how you would behave, how you might describe the situation to a person involved in the scenario or how you would interpret the issues the scenario presents. In general, these mini interviews are designed to evaluate your professionalism, communication skills, ability to work with a team, compassion, and ability to consider all aspects of a situation. Since this type of interview is becoming increasingly more common in the US, and because this style of interview is distinctive, an entire section of the book will be devoted to it.

CHAPTER 3

BEFORE THE INTERVIEW: PRACTICAL CONCERNS

While I realize that some of the content in this chapter might seem elementary, an interview book wouldn't be complete without it!

TRAVEL PLANNING

If you are traveling to a different state for your interview, start making your travel arrangements as soon as you set your interview date. This way, if you must travel by air (be sure to carry on your bag), you are likely to get the best fares. Most medical schools have rolling admissions so it is advisable to schedule your interview at the earliest possible date. Some schools are also starting to offer "virtual interviews" or alumni interviews. My advice is to avoid these alternative options until they become more commonplace and only if people become more comfortable with them. Before you make your plans, it also is advisable to contact schools to which you have applied in the same geographic area where you are interviewing. It is perfectly acceptable to call an admissions office and say: "I am interviewing at a medical school close to yours on October 17th and I am trying to economize. I am really interested in your medical school and I was wondering if a decision has been made on my application." Though many students feel this is pushy, as long as you are respectful, this strategy actually has the advantage of communicating that you are a desirable candidate since you have other interviews, probably moving your application to "the top of the pile," and it allows you to express your interest in the school. Many MedEdits' students have had success using this approach to earn more interview invitations while making the process more efficient. It is fine if your parents, significant other, or a close friend drives you to the interview since this may alleviate your anxiety, but they should not go to the interview with you. Send them to lunch, perhaps, and tell them you will call them (after you have left the vicinity of the medical complex) once you are finished.

Even if the interview day is supposed to end by 2 PM, do not schedule return flights, trains, or rides anytime close to this time. Interviewers may be late and your day may go longer than expected. It is best to make evening travel plans if you are leaving the area the same day as your interview.

Remember that interview season runs from September/October to March/April at most schools so you may well run into winter travel delays. To allow for inclement weather, try not to bunch up interviews too closely together. If you anticipate delays based on a weather prediction, be sure to call the school to let them know about the situation. This communicates that you are reliable and plan ahead.

SLEEP

Obviously, you should try to get a good night's sleep the night before your interview. But pre-interview anxiety may make this difficult. For this reason, I advise applicants to get a full eight hours of sleep for the entire week before an interview, making it less likely that one night of sleep deprivation will negatively impact your performance. IF you don't sleep well the night before your interview, do not stress. The excitement of interview day will carry you through; however, don't be surprised if you crash when it's over!

SHOULD YOU STAY WITH A HOST STUDENT?

Many clients ask me about the pros and cons of staying with a host student. A host should not, in theory, have any influence on your candidacy so this concern should not affect your decision about whether to accept the offer. I suggest doing what will make you most comfortable and help ensure a good night's sleep the night before your interview. For me, staying with a stranger would not be the ideal way to ease anxiety, but this is an individual choice. If you do choose to stay with a host, be respectful; you are a guest in the host's home. In the unlikely event that a host has an influence on your application, keep your conversations a bit more formal than those you would have with a friend; don't say anything negative or tell your host anything you wouldn't want the admissions office to know! If finances are an issue, an alternative would be to stay with a friend or family who lives in the area.

PLAN TO ARRIVE TO YOUR INTERVIEW AT LEAST 15 MINUTES EARLY

If the school instructs you to arrive for your interview at 9 AM, be there at 8:30 or 8:45 at the latest. Make provisions for rush hour traffic, especially if you are in a city. If you are in a new place, it is also wise to do a "dry run" to the medical school so you know exactly where you are going and how to get there. Academic medical complexes are large and often difficult to navigate. If you are late for any reason, be sure to call the admissions office (you will, of course, have the phone number on hand) and let them know.

EAT BREAKFAST!

Even though some schools may have some pastries or bagels when you arrive, you would be wise to eat a healthy breakfast before your interview, making sure to include some protein and to avoid a high-carbohydrate meal so your blood sugar doesn't plummet while you are interviewing (you will learn more about the pathophysiology of this suggestion during medical school). It is okay to drink some coffee the morning of your interview, but if you are especially anxious consider having only a small cup or skipping the caffeine entirely.

PARTICIPATE IN "OPTIONAL" ACTIVITIES

Nothing on the interview day agenda should be considered optional. It is essential to demonstrate interest in the school, so opting out of going to classes, for example, communicates that you aren't serious about the school. While such choices do not affect your evaluation, like everything else, your choices send an overall message about you and your level of enthusiasm for the school and the process. Participating in every activity offered to you also demonstrates respect for the process.

CANCELING INTERVIEWS

It is acceptable to cancel interviews, and most schools expect cancelations late in the season. Be sure to call the medical school admissions office at least two weeks before your interview to cancel and send an email to confirm the cancelation. Canceling interviews is actually a good deed since your interview spot will be offered to another deserving applicant. You do not need to give a reason for canceling. No-shows and "night-before" cancelations are unacceptable.

CHAPTER 4

INTERVIEW DAY: THE NITTY GRITTIES

WHAT TO WEAR

Consider this your first professional job interview and dress accordingly. By "looking the part," you demonstrate respect for the process, the profession, and for the people who are taking time from their day to interview you. If the weather is cold or it is raining, it is acceptable to wear appropriate gear. You will be given a space to keep your belongings. Above all, I encourage students to be comfortable; while you can't wear your sweatpants, the more comfortable you are, the more confident you will be. And remember, it's not a fashion show!

For example, I recently had an applicant who asked me if she should wear her long hair in a bun. When I asked her if she typically wore this hair style, she said, "I have no idea how to put my hair in a bun. A doctor suggested I do this to look more serious." I advised this student to style her hair as she normally does so she has one fewer thing to worry about on interview day. If possible, bring an extra blouse/shirt or some stain remover for last minute emergencies.

WOMEN

Medical school applicants sometimes ask me if they can take purses or shoulder bags to interviews. I am always amazed when I read admissions books that suggest women should take only briefcases to interviews or must wear skirts. (see: What to bring). I think this advice is antiquated and dates back to the 1940s. It is perfectly okay to bring a purse, but don't carry your life's possessions with you; smaller is better. Women should wear a pant or skirt suit. The color does not matter as long as the look is professional. Some women wrongly think they must avoid color completely. As long as you are professional, color is okay and can help you stand out from the "sea of navy blue." In fact, I wore a professional red skirt with a more traditionally colored jacket to my medical school interviews. This felt empowering, and boosted my confidence, but these are individual choices. Avoid low cut shirts, short skirts, and high heels! Wear conservative jewelry and makeup and comfortable closed-toe shoes (no sandals or open-toe). If you are wearing hose, bring an extra pair.

Most physicians do not wear perfume since patients may have allergies, so it is best to leave scent at home. Polished nails can offer a tailored look, but the color should be neutral and your nails should be short. This is not the place for black nail polish. Many women who are married ask if they should wear a ring. You should do what makes you comfortable.

MEN

Since men have fewer choices, this paragraph is short! It is best to wear a dark suit, but colorful ties are welcome! If you have long hair, consider a cut, and I suggest removing any earrings. Many people in medicine are still very conservative so, should you choose to wear an earring or long hair, just be aware of this. It is important to wear comfortable shoes since you will be walking a lot. Be sure to shave before your interview, but leave the aftershave at home. Be neat, tidy, and professional.

REMEMBER....

Overall, how you carry yourself typically is more important than what you wear. The person in the high end suit who seems insecure and lacks confidence will not make as good an impression as the individual who shows up with a slightly wrinkled blouse, scuffed shoes, and unruly hair, yet is self-assured and exudes enthusiasm and intelligence.

WHAT TO BRING:

HAVE SOME CASH FOR INCIDENTALS

I will never forget the applicant who asked us for money to buy a subway token. Enough said.

BRING A SNACK AND A BOTTLE OF WATER

Just in case you unexpectedly have to wait for your interviewer and you become hungry, it is wise to have handy something small and inconspicuous like a granola bar. Interview days can be long and you will be talking a bunch! Therefore, consider toting a water bottle with you.

I find that many medical school applicants are concerned about what they should bring to interviews.

DO NOT BRING A LARGE BACKPACK TO CARRY AROUND WITH YOU

It is too bulky. If you must have a backpack with you because of traveling logistics, plan to ask the admissions office if you can leave it there while you are on your tour and interviews.

IT IS ACCEPTABLE TO BRING A SUITCASE, IF NECESSARY

You can ask where to leave your luggage during your interview. When I interviewed applicants, this situation was commonplace.

BRING A PEN AND FOLDER OR PORTFOLIO

You should take notes during program or school presentations, so be prepared. Most programs will give you folders with literature about the school/program. Do not take notes during your actual interview(s).

BRING ANY RECENT PUBLICATIONS OR UPDATES FOR YOUR INTERVIEWERS

If you have any recent publications, feel free to bring them to hand to the secretary so they can be added to your file. You can also bring extra copies for your interviewers in case they are interested.

BRING THE APPROPRIATE OUTERWEAR

If you are traveling to a cold climate in the middle of the winter, be prepared. If you wear boots because it is snowing, be sure to bring shoes to which you can change. Similarly, if it is raining, wear appropriate gear. Admissions offices have places to store your belongings.

BRING SOMETHING TO READ

Since you will likely have some down time, it is acceptable to bring a book. While I would stay away from romance novels and lightweight magazines, you do not need to bring a medical journal with you. Fiction or the newspaper are good choices and may even spark some discussion. It's best not to scroll on your phone while waiting in any area where you might be "seen."

CHAPTER 5

INTERVIEW DAY TOURS AND LUNCHES

GENERAL

Many clients ask me about how to behave on tours and lunches during interview days. The bottom line is: Always be respectful, open, and kind. Whether you are interacting with a secretary, admissions director, or the person who takes away the trash, it is essential to treat everyone well. Making a strong impression can help you if that impression is positive or hurt you if it is negative. How you treat the support staff is crucial; it says a lot about your character, and even a hint of entitlement or rudeness can significantly hinder your success. I always paid attention to how applicants treated others they met, especially those they might have deemed "unimportant" in the process. This told me volumes about character.

Pretend you are in a fish bowl during your medical school interview day. If you are friendly and personable to all, it can only help your candidacy and affect the overall impression that people have of you.

Be sure to turn off your cell phone, and do not check email during your interview day. You must appear attentive and undistracted the entire day.

TOURS

On tours, be front and center, pay attention, and make eye contact to demonstrate that you are doing so. When I was a tour guide, I could always tell who was lingering, chatting, or was disinterested, and who was really paying attention to what I said. While it is good to ask questions, don't dominate or interrupt the tour guide.

BE KIND TO OTHER APPLICANTS

You will be under the microscope throughout your medical school interview day and constantly being observed. If you are friendly and personable to all, it can only help your candidacy and favorably affect the overall impression that people have of you. Don't spend your time talking about other schools and comparing notes.

LUNCH

Avoid caffeinated beverages during lunch if you are nervous. Demonstrate good table manners. Also, never chew gum, though it is okay to bring breath mints with you. Do not eat a large lunch if your interviews follow the meal as this may make you sleepy.

DON'T...EVER...

Talk negatively about another medical school, a person, applicant, or your undergraduate school.

CHAPTER 6

INTERVIEW ETIQUETTE

YOUR OVERALL DEMEANOR AND NONVERBAL COMMUNICATION

Think about someone who has made a positive impression on you instantly. What qualities did he or she possess? Most likely, he was open, warm, and confident (but not overconfident). It is important to be poised, receptive (smile when you can to show this), and engaging. Be sure your body language conveys these elements, too. Make eye contact. Smile and be friendly. Don't ever slouch and be interested in everyone you meet. In other words, project a degree of professionalism that will distinguish you from your peers. Your nonverbal communication will not be consciously assessed, but every interviewer and person you meet will perceive you based on nonverbal cues. Be aware of your expressions, too. Leave any eye rolling or glaring judgmental looks at home. Practice by watching yourself in the mirror while having conversations. What do you project? Ask others how they generally perceive you and request honesty. Sometimes we are not aware of how we project and what others instinctively perceive about us.

GREETING PEOPLE

Make eye contact with and introduce yourself to everyone you meet and smile naturally! Never call anyone by his or her first name; use his or her title and last name. It always irritated me a bit when an applicant called me by my first name in an initial meeting. If you aren't sure of the person's title, it is always safe to start off with "Dr. XX." Do not extend your hand when you meet someone; instead let her take this initiative since she is senior to you. Have your right hand free so you are prepared and shake hands firmly if presented with this opportunity. Respect the personal space of everyone you meet. Throughout your interview day, be sure to speak at a normal pace, with clear diction, in a normal tone and volume, and in a formal conversational manner. Speaking informally or using slang words anytime during the interview day puts you at risk for being perceived in the wrong way (see, Interview day tours and lunches: How to behave).

IN THE OFFICE

As you enter someone's office, allow her to suggest where you should sit. If she doesn't, wait for her to sit down first and then sit across from her where it seems most natural. Sit up straight and do not slouch. Place anything you are holding on the floor beside you. If you aren't sure what to do with your hands, fold them comfortably into your lap. It is okay to use gestures while you converse, but don't go overboard. Do not forget to smile and try to appear positive, energetic, enthusiastic, and warm. Be sure to make eye contact with your interviewer throughout the interview, especially when she is talking. This demonstrates that you are attentive. This behavior will make your interviewer like you—a primary goal. Do not be offended if your interviewer's pager or cell phone goes off and she needs to answer a call. This is medicine and things come up.

CLOSING THE TRADITIONAL INTERVIEW

When it is obvious that your interview is over, allow your interviewer to stand up first and then you stand up and grab any belongings. Allow your interviewer to continue to the door first and then follow him. He will likely say something like, "I enjoyed meeting you. Do you know how to get to where you need to go?" You should respond: "Thank you for your time. I would be thrilled to come here for medical school and, yes, I know where I am going." Since your interviewer now feels acquainted with you personally, he may give you a mentor-like "pat" or extend his hand for a handshake. Again, pay attention and follow your interviewer's lead. An MMI interview will end differently, and   that ending could feel abrupt since there is a strict time schedule to follow. Don't allow this to unnerve you. MMI raters are not supposed to show any emotion.

FOLLOWING UP AFTER THE INTERVIEW

Write thank you notes or emails for any traditional interviews. They are unlikely to influence your candidacy, but it is good manners to write these notes. Make the note short and sweet and mention anything that was a highlight of your interview; also repeat that you are interested in the school and thank the interviewer for her time. Sometimes admissions offices give applicants suggestions for contacting their interviewers so, if they do, be sure to follow their directions. But wait until you get home to send your thank you notes. I remember the candidate who was writing her thank you notes in the conference room during interview day. She handed them to the secretary before she left. This seemed contrived and insincere. I encourage applicants to write emails instead of written notes. Why? An interviewer will have the chance to respond to an email and a written note is a "one way street" and cannot elicit a reply. However, do not be concerned if an interviewer doesn't hit the reply button to your thank you email. It means nothing!!!! It is not expected that you will follow up after an MMI interview day, however. Only do so if you felt true rapport with someone whom you met.

PART 2:

THE TRADITIONAL MEDICAL SCHOOL INTERVIEW

CHAPTER 7

WHAT IS THE INTERVIEWER LOOKING FOR?

It is important to understand what interviewers are looking for within the context of your experience. Medical school applicants often fail to make a good impression when they try to tell interviewers what they think they want to hear instead of representing themselves honestly and authentically. Since your grades, MCAT scores and letters of reference will be used to evaluate your academic aptitude, interviewers are trying to assess something else-- if you are genuinely committed to a career in medicine and have an understanding of what it means to practice medicine, if you have compassion, empathy, and maturity, your intelligence, and how good your interpersonal and communication skills are— among other attributes. (See Box: What qualities and characteristics do interviewers evaluate? on page 47) Interviewers also want to rule out any red flags, such as gaps in time on your record, many changes in careers or interests or any signs of personal instability.

DO YOU HAVE A DEMONSTRATED COMMITMENT TO AND UNDERSTANDING OF A CAREER IN MEDICINE?

Interviewers are trying to assess first and foremost your motivation to pursue a career in medicine. They want to hear about when and why you want to practice medicine, and they want to know that your background justifies your claim that you want to practice medicine. They also want to know that you understand what you are getting yourself in to and that you understand the pros and cons of practicing medicine and have a realistic idea of the challenges you will face in medicine. This is why some interviewers ask about health care reform; they don't expect you to have an advanced degree in health policy, but they want to know that you at least have some idea of what the issues in health care are today.

ARE YOU CONFIDENT YET HUMBLE?

Even a hint of arrogance or self-righteousness might destroy your chances of acceptance. Humility is much preferred over self-centeredness and a fine line sometimes differentiates confidence from overconfidence. Be sure not to do anything that might suggest you are over confident, for example by acting too informal or familiar, appearing too comfortable, dropping names or obviously promoting yourself. Let your accomplishments speak for themselves and hope that your letter writers wrote about your positive qualities and attributes.

DO YOU HAVE WHAT IT TAKES TO MAKE IT THROUGH MEDICAL SCHOOL, RESIDENCY TRAINING AND A FUTURE MEDICAL CAREER?

It takes a tremendous amount of dedication, resilience and perseverance not only to succeed in medical school but also to do well in residency training, which can be very rigorous. While interviewers will glean information about your strengths based on what is written in your letters of reference, they are also trying to assess these qualities during your interview. A medical education and career pose intellectual, emotional, and physical challenges that a medical school applicant cannot appreciate. So, it is your interviewer's job to decide if you have the characteristics that make it likely you will be able to cope and succeed throughout your medical education.

CAN YOU RECOGNIZE YOUR FAULTS AND ADMIT WHEN YOU ARE WRONG?

No one expects you to be perfect. In fact, admissions committee members want to know that you can recognize your faults and that you can make improvements or modify your behaviors. Did you do poorly in your early years of college and can you explain why? Admissions committees want to know that you can learn from mistakes and that you won't crumble if things don't go as planned. If you had an institutional action during college, admissions committee members want to see that you are remorseful and that you have learned and grown from the experience. They also want to know that you are aware of your limitations. An important part of being a great doctor is knowing when it is time to ask for help and to be aware of your own strengths, expertise, and weaknesses.

IS EVERYTHING CONSISTENT?

Interviewers also want to make sure that what you have written in your application and how you present yourself "match." Misrepresentation in either your application or your interview makes a negative impression. This is also why it's important to write your own personal statement and application! Consistency in your story is key, even if an interview is closed file, and interviewers will try to identify themes in your background and during your interview. Once your interview evaluation is done, it will be "compared," to a degree, with your written application.

ARE YOU SMART AND INTELLECTUALLY CURIOUS?

You also are being evaluated on your intelligence and intellectual curiosity and your ability to think logically and critically. While you won't be asked academic questions, a skilled interviewer can assess your abilities based on how you reason through the questions that are asked.

WHAT IS YOUR DEMEANOR AND
HOW DO YOU COMMUNICATE?

Medical school applicants are judged on whether they are articulate, poised, enthusiastic and mature, can manage difficult questions with ease, and demonstrate empathy and compassion. The best applicants smile, make good eye contact and are engaging, interesting and warm. Be sure you aren't swayed by a negative interviewer. You should greet even the grouchy interviewer happily and warmly and not allow him to "bring you down." People with "sparkling personalities" always do better on interviews than their more sullen, stone faced, or negative peers. Interviewees are also judged on their accomplishments, life experiences, ability to overcome obstacles, and their suitability for a career in medicine. Since communication skills, great interpersonal skills, and the ability to relate to people are necessary to practice medicine, you may be dinged if your interviewer thinks you have difficulty in these areas.

ARE YOU CULTURALLY COMPETENT?

As our country becomes more diverse, physicians must be able to care for individuals of different cultures, religions, races, and socioeconomic backgrounds. This does not mean that admissions committees want to know that you speak a second language; rather, they want to know that you have experience working with people who are different from you and that you are sensitive to the impact of these differences. Can you communicate with patients who have diverse backgrounds? Will you understand how these differences affect patients' compliance and perception of disease, and will you consider a patient's home and community environment when designing your treatment plan?

HOW WILL YOU ADD TO THE MEDICAL SCHOOL'S COMMUNITY?

Your interviewer also will evaluate how you will add to the learning environment and the diversity of the medical school. With the recent emphasis on a holistic review of applicants, this definition of diversity is broad and relates not only to your cultural and racial background but also to your interests and experiences. Most medical school interviewers are open minded and thus hope to attract a broad range of students to their school who can make a valuable and meaningful contribution to the medical community.

ARE YOU A GOOD "FIT" FOR THE MEDICAL SCHOOL?

Schools also are seeking out applicants who are the best fit for their school. For example, a smaller community-focused school may not be interested in the applicant with 10 original publications who wants to make research a part of her career. So, while one applicant may be the ideal student for one school, she may not be the best fit for another. You therefore should study each school's website before you interview to have a sense of what it values, its mission statement, and what kind of students it is trying to attract. As already emphasized, who you are on interview day must match the person the admissions committee reads (or will read) about in your application, but you can often spin your experiences a bit to conform to their ideal student and applicant.

DO YOU HAVE ANY RED FLAGS?

The two most obvious red flags are gaps in time of longer than three months when you cannot account for your activities or frequent jumps in career without any real explanation for these changes. Both of these factors suggest a lack of commitment or some possible underlying problem. Students who cannot communicate or are extremely nervous or anxious also raise concern. Interviewers are also trying to identify any major personality disorder or psychopathology that may hinder a candidate's ability not only to interact with patients and colleagues but the ability to get through medical school and residency. Other common "red flags" include a low grade, GPA, or MCAT score, or an institutional action or withdrawals from classes, but, typically, if you were invited for an interview, these issues were not considered major. That said, you should be able to give explanations for the flaws in your application without making excuses.

HAVE YOU OVERCOME ANY SIGNIFICANT HARDSHIP OR ADVERSITY?

Students who have overcome significant obstacles such as coming from an underserved area, having financial hardship, or being the first in their family to go to college are typically evaluated within the context of this cohort of applicants. Since achieving success with few resources is a tremendous accomplishment, students who have overcome adversity are looked upon favorably because achieving under difficult circumstances requires perseverance, drive, and a true commitment. Also, people who come from underserved areas are more likely to serve such communities in the future, which is why it is in society's best interest (and the medical school's) to attract such applicants.

WHAT ELEMENT OF DIVERSITY DO YOU CONTRIBUTE?

Medical schools now emphasize a holistic review of applicants so they have a broad definition of diversity as mentioned above. Admissions committees are looking for students with a diverse mix of experiences, backgrounds, and perspectives. This does not mean that being a traditional student is a liability. In fact, being traditional (meaning that you haven't had a prior career or come from an underprivileged background) also has advantages because traditional applicants typically present no red flags and are highly motivated and directed. But the applicant who had a prior career or who is an immigrant, for example, also brings diversity to a medical school class. What is important to understand is that every applicant brings an element of diversity regardless of background and experience.

WOULD THE INTERVIEWERS ENJOY SPENDING LONG PERIODS OF TIME WITH YOU?

Since your interviewers see you not only as a medical student candidate but also as a potential future colleague, they want to know that you are, bottom line, good company. So, you must convey that "having you around" would be comfortable and pleasant. This is why small talk matters during your interview day; interviewers want to know that you are personable. It is also important to stay as positive as you can during an interview. Don't complain and stay away from negative comments.

ARE YOU SEXIST OR RACIST?

Any hint that you are biased, closed minded or insensitive will make interviewers check the "rejection" box. I remember how one applicant, when speaking of caring for an inner city population, said, "I have concerns about taking care of people who are underserved. I have never worked with those types of people before." While this comment may have been innocent, it struck the interviewer the wrong way, and she rejected this applicant.

WHAT QUALITIES AND CHARACTERISTICS DO INTERVIEWERS EVALUATE?

Commitment to medicine

Understanding of medicine

Motivation to pursue a career in medicine

Clinical exposure and experience (such as shadowing)

Intellectual abilities

Intellectual curiosity

Scholarly interests

Level of compassion

Level of empathy

Level of altruism

Maturity

Warmth

Professionalism

Cultural competence

Resilience and perseverance

Experience in research

Experience in teaching

Community service experience

Work with underserved populations

Leadership ability

Ability to think critically and analytically

Ability to communicate

Ability to listen

Ability to answer difficult questions

Ability to work as a member of a team

Personality and overall disposition

Reactions to situations (Do you ever become impatient or react impulsively?)

Values

Ability to overcome obstacles and cope with adversity

Achievements that make you stand out

Level of initiative

Red flags

CHAPTER 8

CORE COMPETENCIES IN MEDICAL SCHOOL ADMISSIONS

The Association of American Medical Colleges has identified 15 core competencies that are essential for each medical student. These competencies will also be identified though your written documents and letters of reference. When interviewing you, whether "traditionally," in a group, or through the MMI format, interviewers are assessing you for these qualities, characteristics, and abilities:

1. Service Orientation: Demonstrates a desire to help others and sensitivity to others' needs and feelings; demonstrates a desire to alleviate others' distress; recognizes and acts on his/her responsibilities to society; locally, nationally, and globally.
2. Social Skills: Demonstrates an awareness of others' needs, goals, feelings, and the ways that social and behavioral cues affect peoples' interactions and behaviors; adjusts behaviors appropriately in response to these cues; treats others with respect.
3. Cultural Competence: Demonstrates knowledge of socio-cultural factors that affect interactions and behaviors; shows an appreciation and respect for multiple dimensions of

diversity; recognizes and acts on the obligation to inform one's own judgment; engages diverse and competing perspectives as a resource for learning, citizenship, and work; recognizes and appropriately addresses bias in themselves and others; interacts effectively with people from diverse backgrounds.

4. Teamwork: Works collaboratively with others to achieve shared goals; shares information and knowledge with others and provides feedback; puts team goals ahead of individual goals.

5. Oral Communication: Effectively conveys information to others using spoken words and sentences; listens effectively; recognizes potential communication barriers and adjusts approach or clarifies information as needed.

6. Ethical Responsibility to Self and Others: Behaves in an honest and ethical manner; cultivates personal and academic integrity; adheres to ethical principles and follows rules and procedures; resists peer pressure to engage in unethical behavior and encourages others to behave in honest and ethical ways; develops and demonstrates ethical and moral reasoning.

7. Reliability and Dependability: Consistently fulfills obligations in a timely and satisfactory manner; takes responsibility for personal actions and performance.

8. Resilience and Adaptability: Demonstrates tolerance of stressful or changing environments or situations and adapts effectively to them; is persistent, even under difficult situations; recovers from setbacks.

9. Capacity for Improvement: Sets goals for continuous improvement and for learning new concepts and skills; engages in reflective practice for improvement; solicits and

responds appropriately to feedback.

10. Critical Thinking: Uses logic and reasoning to identify the strengths and weaknesses of alternative solutions, conclusions, or approaches to problems.

11. Quantitative Reasoning: Applies quantitative reasoning and appropriate mathematics to describe or explain phenomena in the natural world.

12. Scientific Inquiry: Applies knowledge of the scientific process to integrate and synthesize information, solve problems, and formulate research questions and hypotheses; is facile in the language of the sciences and uses it to participate in the discourse of science and explain how scientific knowledge is discovered and validated.

13. Written Communication: Effectively conveys information to others using written words and sentences.

14. Living Systems: Applies knowledge and skill in the natural sciences to solve problems related to molecular and macro systems, including biomolecules, molecules, cells, and organs.

15. Human Behavior: Applies knowledge of the self, others, and social systems to solve problems related to the psychological, socio-cultural, and biological factors that influence health and well-being.

CHAPTER 9

WHO WILL INTERVIEW YOU?

Most interviews are conversational and biographical. You may be interviewed by admissions deans and directors, administrators in the admissions office, clinical faculty (the MD type), basic science faculty (the PhD type) or medical students.

Always remember that your interviewer is your advocate. She (or he) will "sell you" to the admissions committee. Remember your interviewer is human and, most of the time, is not trying to "get you." She wants to find out about you as a person and if you will be a good fit for the school.

Because your interviewer is the primary support for your candidacy it is essential to get on her good side. Whether she writes up reports or summaries about you or presents you verbally to a committee, your interviewer typically makes or breaks your acceptance. If she thinks highly of you, you're usually in, but if you don't make a good impression, she will not support you. Because you cannot control or predict who will interview you, it is important to have broad appeal as an interviewee and prepare yourself for multiple scenarios.

Considering my experience working with many interviewers and many applicants, I find that the types of interviewers fall into eight general categories, each of which calls for a different candidate approach. The "type" of interviewer you have will influence how a traditional interview proceeds, but, less so for an MMI interview. To direct a traditional interview to your advantage, whether that be open file, closed file, or partially closed file, you need to try early in the interview not only to get a fix on which type of interviewer you have but her perspective and level of experience, which also will affect how your interview progresses. Because most medical school interviewers receive no training in interviewing candidates they do not necessarily know how to evaluate you comprehensively and effectively, as do more experienced interviewers. Why is this important? It is because these inexperienced interviewers (who are most likely to be certain of the types described below) tend to ask more questions and have a different approach than more seasoned interviewers. Feedback from MedEdits applicants has confirmed that students encounter all of these "types" of interviewers.

TYPES OF INTERVIEWERS

THE MENTOR

The mentor is the most common type of interviewer and represents the typical medical educator. These interviewers tend to conduct relaxed yet serious interviews and have a fair amount of experience doing them. Typically, the mentor will ask you basic questions about your background and motivations. These interviewers are confident in their abilities, are committed to medical education, and have extensive experience working with students. They know that the best way to gain the greatest understanding of your motivations, intelligence, and character is if you feel comfortable. Their questions therefore tend to be basic and predictable. Fortunately, most medical school interviewers are mentors, and, in general, the interviews they conduct are "easy." Indeed, most candidates walk away from these interviews feeling confident and thinking, "That interviewer really liked me." But, it's important not to become too comfortable and informal during these interviews simply because you feel confident that you are making a good impression. Remember that while the interviewer is your advocate, he is not your friend.

THE PROFESSOR

These interviewers can, based on appearance, seem to be the most intimidating when, in reality, they are usually great interviewers. They are very experienced, have worked in different settings, have interviewed many candidates, residents, and attendings, and have a vast amount of experience. They know what they are looking for and how to get the information they need and typically are efficient in seeking it out. Thus, your interview with the professor may veer off in another direction; you may start talking in depth about your research or your interest in philosophy or medical anthropology. Unlike the Question Shooter and the Inappropriate interviewer (see below), however, the professor typically goes off on a tangent because he has effectively and efficiently assessed your candidacy and therefore has time to spare. He is confident in his abilities and is comfortable getting off topic. In some ways, the professor is the interviewer you want; he typically has a strong political voice on admissions committees, and if he supports your candidacy he can be a tremendous advocate. But, the reverse is also true; if he is not in favor of you, his opinion will also weigh heavily.

THE QUESTION SHOOTER

This is most students' worst nightmare. This interviewer might ask you what three people you would like to invite to dinner and why. He may also ask you about your greatest strength and weakness or ask you a very unusual question. Typically, the Question Shooter is inexperienced and asks questions because he fundamentally doesn't know how to interview. He thinks asking random questions is what he is supposed to do and isn't even sure of the answers he is hoping to hear or how to evaluate your response. In some ways, these are the toughest interviews because you can in no way rely on your interviewer to ask you about what you want to tell him. The best way to manage these interviewers is to try to guide the interview. Make segues. Bring up topics you hope to discuss. (How to guide your interview will be discussed again later on in this book.) Some schools have a standard list of questions that they like interviewers to ask candidates. The Question Shooter cannot typically be swayed, however. It is best to try and answer these questions as fully as possible, but don't expect the interviewer to "take the bait" of your segues and direction.

THE INAPPROPRIATE INTERVIEWER

You are unlikely to have this type of interviewer because she usually doesn't last long on admissions committees. Typically, an applicant complains and this interviewer is asked to leave the committee. You can spot an eccentric interviewer by the way she asks you sensitive or even illegal questions, often boring into the most sensitive topic in your background and delving into it. These interviewers think that by "digging" they will gain more information about your character or motivations. Again, the best way to cope with these interviewers is to try and guide your interview and bring up topics you would like to discuss. When asked a question that you think may be illegal, such as about your sexuality, family plans, or religion, it is best to answer vaguely and to try and change the topic. If you are really offended by an interviewer's questions, you should tell the dean of admissions about your experience and request another interview.

THE EGOMANIAC

Ah, the Egomaniacs. They are tough nuts to crack. They are generally young and inexperienced, and they are psyched to be in a position of power. They think they have your life in their hands, and they have told all of their friends that they are on the medical school admissions committee. They proclaim to all that they are important. In some ways, the Egomaniac is the toughest interviewer to impress, and it is not unusual for the Egomaniac to want to hear himself speak as much as he wants to hear you speak. You cannot rely on the egomaniac to ask you about factors that will be relevant to your candidacy so you must guide your interview and be sure to impart the information that you know is important.

THE STRONG SILENT TYPE

The Strong Silent type likes to listen. These interviewers may not ask too many questions. These types are rare since those who are shy do not typically volunteer to be on admissions committees. These interviewers are most challenging for shy applicants, and I envision a very quick interview when they get together. Your major concern if you get a Strong Silent type is that he is unlikely to loudly advocate for you during a medical school admissions committee meeting, so you must hope that the school requires only a written evaluation.

THE SURE, I'LL DO IT TYPE

The Sure, I'll Do It interviewer is the person who was asked by his chairperson to serve on the medical school admissions committee or was pulled in at the last minute when an interviewer was desperately needed. This interviewer is usually participating because he thinks he "should" and may have a relaxed attitude or he may be really annoyed because he had other plans for his day that has now been interrupted because of your interview. Regardless, it is unlikely that he is fully invested in the process. These interviews tend to be fairly relaxed and undirected, but if you get someone who is annoyed, he may take this out on you. The issue with the Sure I'll Do It interviewer is that you must provide him with the information that you know is important. These interviewers may not be the strongest advocates. Thus, it is important to arm them with information about you and your motivations that they otherwise might not ask about.

THE STUDENT INTERVIEWER

Many medical schools encourage current medical students to interview prospective students. But, like their faculty counterparts on the admissions committee, medical students frequently get little or no training on how to interview applicants. When I was on faculty, I thought that having current medical students (and current residents for residency) interview candidates was a great idea since they could judge an applicant's fit for the school. Now that I am privy to hearing about these interviews from the applicant's perspective, however, I think students sometimes lack the experience to make such influential choices. Many applicants tell me, "My interview with the student didn't go so well." I think student interviewers leave this impression because often they don't know what exactly they are seeking. They tend to like concrete answers and often ask many specific questions (like the Question Shooter). They sometimes can become too informal with applicants and end up discussing personal issues and topics that don't relate to the applicant's candidacy. I encourage applicants to approach the student interviewer with the understanding that these interviewers are young and often immature and may not have any experience. Applicants therefore should make sure to approach the student interviewer with a clear idea of their strengths and the aspects of the application that they would like to discuss.

CHAPTER 10

MAKING THE MOST OF THE
TRADITIONAL INTERVIEW

Whatever type of interviewers you have or their level of experience, you can maintain some control of what transpires. (Even the Question Shooter, while difficult to manipulate, can be directed by your responses.) Give complete answers (as a rule, never answer with simply a "yes" or "no") and elaborate. Do not memorize your answers or deliver something "canned." Expect the unexpected. You should try not to ramble, say "um" or "like" too much, fidget in your seat, or display nervous tics. Here are some other general guidelines for making the interview go as well as possible and to make sure that you convey everything that you think is important about your candidacy:

BE AUTHENTIC

This may seem simple, but interviewees who are "comfortable in their own skin" stand out versus applicants who try to say what they think everyone wants to hear. Even if your interviewer isn't specifically evaluating you on your authenticity, an applicant who speaks the truth in his own words typically exudes confidence and professionalism. Sometimes the most distinctive applicants are those who are the most natural and possess a true sense of themselves. Authenticity is also important for an MMI interview!

MAKE A GOOD FIRST IMPRESSION

Even if it is subconscious, your interviewer makes a judgment about you within the first five to 10 minutes of your interview regardless of the type of interview. If the interviewer has a positive impression, this "halo effect" will affect everything you say. Similarly, an initial negative impression (the "horns effect") will also cast a shadow and it will be tough to redeem yourself. Making a good first impression is based not only on what you say but on your general demeanor. Are you professional, poised, energetic, positive, and enthusiastic? The impression you convey in the first few minutes by your overall attitude, energy, tone of voice, and expression will set the stage for everything that follows. Remember never to say anything negative during an interview about other schools or people, which may give a poor impression.

Even small talk at the appropriate time can have an important effect, either positive or negative. You might find yourself speaking with a member of the faculty or a current student who is not interviewing you before the school presentation, for example. If this person has a strong impression of you, whether positive or negative, she will likely express it when your candidacy is discussed.

CREATE YOUR OWN AGENDA

By agenda, I mean an outline in your mind (you don't want to display a crib sheet) of the key things about you and your experiences that you would like to discuss. This is essential because you cannot rely on your interviewer to ask about everything you would like to discuss, even all of your key experiences; you must take responsibility for bringing them up even if you wrote about them in your application. Remember that even if an interview is open file, your interviewer may not have had the time to review your materials. Also, think about how your experiences and values are similar to the mission and philosophy of the school to which you are applying. Be sure to speak about your experiences in this context. In any type of "traditional" one on one interview, you will have the opportunity to guide the interview to a degree. You can do this by mentioning things you would like to discuss further. Most interviews are conversational so, if you really want to talk about your upbringing in another state, mention this in some context. Similarly, if you really want to discuss your recent research or shadowing experience, bring that up at some point during your interview. We always encourage applicants to know what their most distinguishing experiences, qualities, and insights are before they go in to interviews. Often it takes an outside objective party (like a MedEdits faculty member) to identify what aspects of your background and characteristics are most compelling!

MAKE THE INTERVIEWER'S JOB EASY

When I interviewed applicants, the most painful interviews made me feel that getting information from an applicant was "like pulling teeth." In contrast, the easiest interviews were with candidates who had a lot to say that was pertinent and important. These interviewees were obviously better prepared, which impressed me because it indicated that they were taking the interview seriously enough to practice. Even though I was never a Question Shooter, the applicants who gave brief answers forced me to dip into my "interview questions bank" since they said so little. Ideally, you should make your interviewer's job easy by providing her with insights and anecdotes and making segues. You don't want to ramble, but as long as you stick to the agenda you've created, it's most likely that you will gravitate to pertinent topics while making things simpler for your interviewer.

MAKE SEGUES AND GIVE COMPLETE ANSWERS

Again, this comes back to the idea that you are in control. Make segues to topics you would like to discuss. For example, if you are asked why you want to be a doctor, explain not only "why" but "when" and "what." Tell the interviewer when your interest started and what you have done to explore it. By the same token, if you are asked "what is your most valuable volunteer experience" tell the interviewer not only "what" and "when" but also "why" and "how" you became interested in this activity. If you practice doing this, your segues should become natural and conversational, and your interviewer will remain engaged in what you are saying. By making these references and elaborating, you will naturally inspire further discussion and create prompts for your interviewer. This is why it is important to know what your "agenda" is as well as your most important experiences. With this in mind, you can try to make segues and mentions to talk about what is most important to you and most distinguishing about you.

DON'T RELY ON YOUR INTERVIEWER!

This sounds odd to a medical school applicant, but, repeats ideas already mentioned. No one knows you, your experiences, what distinguishes you, and what makes you a great applicant better than YOU do!!! Therefore, know your application, your most valuable experiences, viewpoints, and curiosities and bring those subjects up during your interview even if your interviewer does not!

TRY YOUR BEST TO MAKE YOUR INTERVIEW CONVERSATIONAL

The more experienced interviewers will naturally try to make your interview conversational but, just like any conversation, your interview is a give and take so do your best to keep the flow going. At the same time, be sure that you keep an air of formality to your interview even if your interviewer becomes too informal. Also, try not to dwell too much on one topic or to get off topic. Unless the interviewer is a dean of admissions or someone who is very experienced and has already covered many of the basics of your experience and motivations, you should make it your job not to allow the interview to get off track. This usually is a risk only with an inexperienced interviewer.

BRING UP "RED FLAGS"

Be sure to strategically bring up any possible "red flags," but don't dwell on them. Don't make excuses for any flaws in your application. Explain why they happened succinctly, and be straightforward and matter of fact. You may think that it would be ideal if the interviewer doesn't bring up a red flag in your application, such as gaps in time or a very low MCAT score or grades. In reality, it is best if you have an opportunity to address these issues during the interview because they inevitably will come up in behind-the-scenes discussions about you and, if your interviewer is not armed with an explanation, he will not be in a position to defend you. This puts you at a disadvantage. Here are some common red flags:

1) LOW GPA OR MCAT

First of all, if you've made it to the interview stage, your GPA and MCAT were "good enough!" That said, it is most likely you had a poor year or maybe you didn't do so well as an undergraduate and then "proved" yourself in a special master's program. Many students don't do well early in college because they don't have the proper study skills, maturity, or focus. No one is perfect, and it is important to be honest about your flaws and why you underperformed. Maybe you were going through a tough time because a family member was sick, or your parents were getting divorced. It's best to disclose what might have contributed to a low GPA while, at the same time, explaining what you did to then improve your academic performance. Was your first MCAT score very low and did you then bump your score? What did you do to improve that score?

2) NOT HAVING A LONG STANDING COMMITMENT TO MEDICINE

Some applicants did not realize they wanted to go to medical school until later in college or after college. Again, honesty is best. Not everyone has know since kindergarten that he or she wants to be a doctor. Be honest about your path. Explain when and why you became interested in medicine if you think your commitment might not be so obvious.

INSTITUTIONAL ACTION OR MISDEMEANOR

Honesty is always the best policy when discussing any possible poor judgment that may have happened in the past. Discuss what happened, succinctly, and explain what you then did to remediate and improve. Show remorse and understanding for your actions. It is most important to discuss what you learned from the situation. Everyone is allowed to make mistakes. What is often most important is how you react to that mistake and the steps you take moving forward.

TALKING FOR TOO LONG

Keep in mind that your interviewer's attention span is short. Don't speak for longer than three minutes about any one topic unless you sense that your interviewer wants to hear more. Pay attention to body language and cues; do you sense that your interviewer wants to interrupt you and ask a question? Does he look bored--should you wrap up your answer and allow your interviewer to move you to another topic? Is he making eye contact and acting engaged in what you are saying? There are no absolute rules for how long you should speak; it all depends on the dynamics of your actual interview.

INTERVIEWING THE INTERVIEWER

Do not turn the interview around on your interviewer and start asking her questions about her career and motivations unless this happens naturally. This can be interpreted as disrespectful or make the interviewer "work" when your job is to make hers easy. On the other hand, if an interviewer mentions things about herself or if you share common career interests and goals, it is only natural to ask her questions. This not only demonstrates that you are curious, but it also shows that you have excellent interpersonal skills, both of which are essential to practicing medicine. As with other aspects of the interview, what you discuss should be guided by the individual interviewer and the rapport between the two of you rather than by any firm rules.

Most schools will not identify your interviewer in advance, and I discourage applicants from seeking out this information. Even if the school's policy is to notify applicants in advance about who will interview them, I don't recommend researching your interviewer. Not only are last minute changes common, but interviewers are not concerned about how much applicants know about them. They are more focused on what you know about their school.

REMEMBER, YOU CANNOT BE
PREPARED FOR EVERYTHING

During the first five to seven minutes of your interview you probably will feel anxious or ill at ease. This is normal and will improve as the interview proceeds. Try to anticipate how you respond when you are nervous and alter your behavior accordingly. Listen carefully to the questions your interviewer asks before you respond. But keep in mind that no matter how much you prepare for interviews, unpredictable questions or situations can arise. This is why I encourage applicants to have an understanding of what they want to convey. At the same time, the unexpected question can really throw the applicant who memorizes and over prepares responses. To keep interviewing interesting for me, every year I prepared one unusual question that I asked all applicants. Inevitably, this question generated some entertaining responses, and I learned unusual things about applicants. I will never forget the applicant whom I asked to teach me something. She got up, saying, "I am going to teach you how to hula hoop." She proceeded to show me the exact way to move my hips. This applicant was outstanding, and her colorful response only enhanced my opinion of her since she had a sense of humor, was confident, and could spontaneously think outside of the box. If you are asked a question that "throws you," however, it is perfectly acceptable to pause and say, "Let me think about that." Most people are not comfortable with silences, but they are okay, and your interviewer will always allow you time to think.

Make sure to close your interview and thank your interviewer. Your interviewer may provide you with an opportunity to make closing remarks, but if he doesn't be sure to make your own opportunity. Close your interview with something strong, sincere, and natural: "I would be honored to matriculate at X for medical school. There is so much about the medical school that I value, and I feel this would be a great fit for me. Thank you so much for taking the time to interview me today." Remember that your interviewer (unless a dean) does not get paid to interview you and volunteers to be on the medical school admissions committee because he enjoys meeting applicants and understands the importance of selecting tomorrow's doctors.

CHAPTER 11

BEHAVIORAL INTERVIEW QUESTIONS

As a part of any traditional interview, you could be posed with behavioral questions. These types of questions assess your reaction to specific situations in your life. In posing these queries, the interview committee is trying to assess your qualities and characteristics in a more significant way. They want to know your reactions to situations, how you cope, how you manage stress, how your perceive situations, and about your values and ideals. As the name suggests, they are tying to figure out how your moral code and qualities influence your behavior. This is important because your past behavior will likely predict your future behavior.

WHAT ARE SOME COMMON
MEDICAL SCHOOL BEHAVIORAL QUESTIONS?

- Tell me about a time you failed.
- Tell me about an obstacle you have overcome.
- Tell me about a time you were part of a team and someone on your team didn't pull his or her weight.
- Tell me about a time you were embarrassed.
- Give me an example of a time you were under extreme pressure and how you dealt with that.

- Give me an example of a time things didn't go as you planned. How did you deal with this?
- Tell me about your most important accomplishment.
- Tell me about a time you were disappointed.
- Tell me about something that irritates you.
- Tell me about a time you failed to communicate effectively.
- Tell me about a time you didn't act professionally.
- Give me an example of when you were disrespectful to someone.
- When was a time you became angry or frustrated?
- When was a time someone disagreed with your actions or views?
- Tell me about a time you made an unpopular decision.
- Tell me about a challenge you encountered.

A GOOD GENERAL APPROACH FOR BEHAVIORAL INTERVIEWS IS TO RESPOND IN THE FOLLOWING WAY:

- Describe the situation in detail. Show you understand all "sides" of the situation.
- As in the MMI, interviewers want to know you can see all sides of a situation clearly and not just your own.
- What were your responses and/or actions to the situation?
- What was the result of your response or actions?
- What did you learn from this?
- What might you have done differently?

Communicating what you learned or what you could have done differently shows you are open to improvement and that you are humble.

Be prepared for follow up questions to anything you say. Remember, all traditional interviews are conversations to an extent. Do not try to have responses prepared for every type of behavioral interview question. Part of what the interviewer is assessing is your ability to think on your feet, your authenticity, humility, compassion, and who you really are with regard to your values and ideals.

CHAPTER 12

HOW SHOULD YOU PREPARE
FOR INTERVIEW DAY?

REVIEW ALL OF YOUR APPLICATION MATERIALS

Anything about which you have written in your application is fair game for discussion. Be sure to review your primary application, secondary application, and any update letters you have sent the school. You must be able to speak articulately about each of your experiences, what you learned from them, and how they led you to and confirmed your interest in medicine. If you have listed any research in your application, be sure you can explain and discuss it intelligently. Also be able to talk about your academic interests and anything you have done since submitting your application.

I strongly discourage applicants from memorizing answers; sounding rehearsed can undermine your authenticity and thus your success. The line between practicing so you are prepared and being over-rehearsed is a fine one. Avoiding sounding "canned" can be especially challenging if you receive multiple interviews and are asked similar questions at all of them.

Be able to speak about any accomplishments or events since you submitted your application. The medical school application process is fluid so you can continue to improve your candidacy after you submit your application.

THINK ABOUT YOUR PATH

The best way to prepare for medical school interviews is to really think about your path and how you got to the seat in which you are sitting on interview day. This may sound simple, but I am always surprised when candidates who obviously have great experiences and have done "all the right things" to get in to medical school cannot connect the dots in their own experience. Think about the overarching themes in your background, when you decided to pursue a career in medicine, and what helped confirm your interest. How has one experience led you to the next? By creating your agenda, you will know your exact path to medicine.

KNOW THE SCHOOL WHERE YOU ARE INTERVIEWING

Since medical schools not only want to find the best applicants but also those who are the best fit for their institution, you must know the details about every school where you interview. Review the school's mission statement, philosophy, curriculum, clinical sites where you will be doing rotations, extracurricular and community service opportunities, and any recent changes they are promoting. Have an idea of what the school is "known for." For example, is it a research focused institution or does it have a great global or public health program? I also suggest that students review the student profiles that some schools have on their websites to get an idea of the types of people they like (since these profiles will likely be the students of whom they are most proud). Also do some research about the area's demographics and geography since that will tell you what's important to the medical school as well. Does the school's primary hospital care for an underserved population? Is it in an urban or rural area? Seeking out information may be easy for private schools, but public schools tend to have websites that are more basic and not as informative. For schools that have less than stellar websites, you should seek out information from current students or rely on interview day to become informed about the school.

PRACTICE!

Most students are not comfortable with the interview process initially although most find it enjoyable as they progress in the interview season. Interviewing well is a skill and it is important that you become comfortable speaking openly about yourself with a stranger. Once you reach the interview stage in the medical school admissions process, it is the most important factor in your success. With more and more emphasis begin placed on an applicant's personal qualities and characteristics, your accomplishments, GPA, and MCAT will not automatically translate to an acceptance regardless of how good they are. Doing mock interviews will not only help you become better at talking about yourself, what's important to you, and what you have accomplished, but it will also help you learn about any distracting habits you may have. What does your body language say about you? How about your expressions? Projecting confidence, but not being overconfident, and making it clear you are open, approachable, and professional during your interview are key. Only with practice will you know if you possess these qualities. With more practice you will also be more confident on interview day.

With whom you practice is very important. Typically, friends and family members may not be well suited to evaluate how you are as an interviewee, and the last thing you want to do is get an opinion from someone is not trained or experienced to evaluate your interview skills. We advise doing mock interviews with your career center or an advisor at school who understands the medical school admissions process well. MedEdits also provides professional mock interview services, and all of our faculty have extensive admissions committee experience. When practicing, always keep in mind that you should not memorize responses or be over rehearsed. Having a natural and organic interview is important and the goal of practice should be to make you more comfortable on interview day so you can be authentic and true to who you are, which will allow you to show your best self.

TYPICAL INTERVIEW SCHEDULE

THE TRADITIONAL INTERVIEW SCHEDULE

Traditional interview days vary but follow a general pattern. Some schools will allow you to go to classes with students, but the schedule generally is similar to the one below.

8:30 AM: Arrive at the interview office
9:00 AM: Presentation by a dean or director of admissions about the school
10:30 AM: Interview #1
12 noon: Lunch

1:00 PM: Interview #2

2:30 PM: School tour conducted by current medical students

THE MMI INTERVIEW SCHEDULE

Like traditional interview days, the MMI interview day will follow a typical pattern.

8:30 AM: Arrive at the interview office

9:00 - 8:45 AM: Welcome and Multiple Mini-Interview (MMI) Overview

8:45 AM: Gather for MMI

9:00 am - 10:45 AM: Multiple Mini-Interview

11:00 am - 11:45 AM: Presentation by a dean or director of admissions

12:00 pm - 2:30 PM Lunch and tour

CHAPTER 13

WHAT HAPPENS AFTER YOU LEAVE?

After the traditional interview day, the admissions committee will meet to formally discuss all applicants. The meeting can happen immediately after the interview, but more typically these meetings are held on a weekly or biweekly basis.

THE WRITTEN SUMMARY

Typically, interviewers fill out a written summary of your candidacy after the interview. They "grade" you on your accomplishments, academics, research, letters of reference, and ability to overcome adversity, among other factors in your candidacy. They also grade you on your personality, enthusiasm, ability to communicate, empathy, compassion, leadership ability, and motivation for a career in medicine. They try to determine if they believe you will do well as a medical student, contribute to the medical community, and would be a good fit for the school. Interviewers may fill this form out immediately after your interview or sometime during the day when they have time. They will likely refer to their notes and your application when completing this form, but how they evaluate you will mostly be based on their overall impression of you.

Sometimes, these forms are submitted to the senior members of the admissions committee, who make a decision about your acceptance, rejection, or wait list status, but more often your interviewer "presents" you at a meeting of all members of the admission committee.

THE VERBAL SUMMARY

Admissions committee meetings are usually held weekly so, for example, if meetings are on Mondays and your interviews were on a Tuesday, your interviewers will each "present you" based on what they have written and on what they remember the following week. The "snapshot" that your interviewers present typically takes no more than five minutes, and they tell the other members of the committee what they suggest should be the decision on your application. Then, all members vote on your candidacy, and the outcome of the vote usually seals the decision. So, you can see that if your interviewers advocate for you, they essentially make the decision about your fate. It does happen that two interviewers disagree about a candidate, and this is when things get interesting. It is also why it is so important to have an interviewer who will really go to bat for you and fight for your candidacy. Some admissions committees allow vetoes, so if a member strongly feels that a candidate should be rejected, this decision cannot be overturned. Ultimately, the dean of admissions makes all decisions and theoretically can overturn a committee decision, but this almost never happens unless some vital piece of information is uncovered after an interview.

WHAT IS A TYPICAL VERBAL "COMMITTEE PRESENTATION"?

"Applicant X is an outstanding young man. He grew up in California and was initially inspired to pursue a career in medicine when his grandfather became ill. He has volunteered in hospitals since high school and has done in depth research. He also is committed to helping the underserved and has volunteered in a free clinic for four years. He graduated from college in May and is spending this year doing oncology research and is likely to be published. He has extensive shadowing, volunteer, and leadership experiences. He did poorly his freshman year with an overall GPA of 3.0 because he was adjusting to college, but he rebounded his sophomore through senior years with a 3.8 average. He has a 512 on his MCAT with an even distribution. His letters of reference are outstanding and support my assessment of him. This young man is sensitive, compassionate, humble, and intellectually curious and is clearly motivated to become a physician scientist. I think he would be a wonderful fit here and he seems sincere about wanting to attend. I think we should take him."

Surprisingly, most committee presentations are brief and boil down your candidacy to a nutshell. And, assuming that all interviewers agree, these committee votes and decisions can be quick!

CHAPTER 14

THE BS/MD INTERVIEW OR EARLY ADMISSION INTERVIEW

Accelerated (6- or 7-year) and early admission medical programs are designed for high school or college students who know they want to pursue careers in medicine. BS/MD programs may involve two sets of interviews; one with the undergraduate college and one with the medical school. For the vast majority of BS/MD programs, the undergraduate college associated with the program will not be as competitive as the medical school; therefore, often these programs do not require an undergraduate interview.

Most early admission and accelerated programs require students to maintain a certain grade point average in their undergraduate course work to keep their position in the medical school. For those that require students to take the MCAT, a minimum MCAT score might also be required. Every year I receive calls from students who were unable to meet this criterion. Typically, students fail to maintain the minimum GPA because they become distracted by social activities, take their medical school seat for granted, or find other interests when they have freedom and are somewhat removed from parental pressure.

Thus, interviewers at these programs are trying to assess several characteristics:

- Are you mature?
- Are you truly committed to a career in medicine, and do
- you understand what it means to be a physician?
- Are you going to "make it?"

Your interviewer wants to be sure that you have the diligence, focus, maturity and discipline to take on a rigorous course load. They also want to know that you are pursuing this path because it is what you want and not because of pressure from your parents. Your interviewer is trying to assess the likelihood that you will succeed if you don't have your parents around to "keep you on track." The path you are taking will not be easy and will require you to work incredibly hard and interviewers need to make sure you realize this. Applicants to BS/MD and early admissions programs and a very accomplished group who have often accomplished as much as the typical premedical applicant. It makes sense, then, that these programs are very competitive and earning an interview is an huge victory in and of itself.

Some interview questions that are unique to BS/MD and early admissions programs:

- What will be the greatest challenges you will face in this program?
- Why do you want to pursue an accelerated program rather than the traditional route to medical school?
- How do you know you want to be a doctor?

- When did you know you wanted to be a doctor?
- What have you done without the influence of your parents?
- How do you manage your time and remember everything you need to do?
- What undergraduate studies interest you?
- How will you manage the pressure of medical school?
- What will you do with "extra time" attending such a program will afford you?
- What motivates you?

CHAPTER 15

THE OSTEOPATHIC MEDICAL SCHOOL INTERVIEW

A majority of osteopathic medical schools conduct traditional interviews, but some have converted to the MMI. In reality, osteopathic interviews do not differ much from allopathic medical school interviews. Therefore, for the most part, there is not a distinctive way to prep for the osteopathic medical school interview.

There are, however, a few things for which students should be prepared and we suggest being able to answer the following questions:

1) WHY OSTEOPATHIC MEDICAL SCHOOL?

Even though osteopathic physicians, for the most part, practice medicine no differently than allopathic physicians, the one major difference in training is that osteopathic medical students learn about manipulative therapy. While many never use these skills in actual practice, you don't want to express that concern during interviews. Instead, if asked "why osteopathic medical school," explain what interests you most about the osteopathic approach.

SAMPLE RESPONSE:

"I appreciate osteopathic medicine's holistic approach to patient care and that doctors really partner with patients to achieve good health. When I shadowed Dr. Carr, I liked how he connected with his patients and helped them adopt workable preventive health care plans. He treated his patients as individuals and worked with each patient within the context of his or her background, culture, and habits. Even though Dr. Carr did not practice manipulative therapy, I am extremely interested in learning about it during medical school."

Whatever happens, do NOT bash allopathic medicine in the process of explaining why the values of osteopathy appeal to you. Also keep in mind that you want to be an osteopathic doctor for the same reasons you want to be an allopathic doctor! You don't need to completely reinvent your responses for osteopathic interview questions. Some of the content will be identical for both types of schools!

2) TELL ME ABOUT YOUR OSTEOPATHIC MEDICINE RELATED ACTIVITIES

All applicants to osteopathic medical schools should have experience shadowing an osteopathic physician. It is tough to convince anyone that you are interested in the discipline if you haven't had any exposure! Be able to discuss all of the osteopathic-related experiences you have had and also discuss any experiences that might be upcoming.

3) ARE YOU ALSO APPLYING TO ALLOPATHIC MEDICAL SCHOOLS?

I find that most students do not get this question; however, if you do, be honest! Explain that you are applying to both types of medical schools if that is the truth. There is no need to justify why you are applying to both allopathic and osteopathic schools. Be matter of fact about it!

What is important is not to make it seem like osteopathic medical schools are your "back up" choice. Be enthusiastic about what you appreciate about the osteopathic approach. I suggest applicants review the AACOM website before interviewing: https://www.aacom.org/become-a-doctor/about-om. Remain positive, do not bash allopathic schools or the allopathic approach, and make it clear that you know the benefits of an osteopathic education and the osteopathic philosophy. Many of our clients tell us that osteopathic interviews focus only on osteopathic medicine and the subject of allopathic medicine and schools does not even come up, so be sure that you don't bring it up if that is the case at your interview!

CHAPTER 16

THE CARIBBEAN MEDICAL SCHOOL INTERVIEW

Caribbean medical school interviews take place in the United States either at a school's US home office or with a graduate of the school. If the interview is conducted at a school office, an administrator typically conducts it. Alumni interviewers may be residents or practicing physicians. Alumni interviewers do not get paid; they are volunteers. Caribbean medical school interviews are usually fairly low stress and consist of basic interview questions. Interviewers are trying to assess your interest in their specific school and want to know that you will be able to cope while studying on a Caribbean island where you will be far away from home and won't have the luxuries to which you may be accustomed. Many people say living on a Caribbean island is often similar to living in a third world country so your interviewer wants to know that you will be able to handle this situation. That said, since Caribbean medical schools are "for profit" and may not have the same limited enrollments as US schools, many interviewers are not overly concerned with these issues since they aren't sacrificing a seat in the class if you "don't make it."

Some specific questions you may be asked on Caribbean medical school interviews:

WHY DO YOU WANT TO GO TO SCHOOL IN THE CARIBBEAN?

For this question, be sure you have researched the school where you will be interviewing. Know the structure of the preclinical curriculum, where you will be rotating in your third year, and where graduates tend to go for residency. You want to demonstrate that you have done your homework and that you are making an informed decision to apply to Caribbean medical schools.

WHAT ARE YOUR EXPECTATIONS OF GOING TO SCHOOL IN THE CARIBBEAN?

WHAT ARE SOME OF THE CHALLENGES YOU ANTICIPATE BY GOING TO SCHOOL HERE?

You will not be going on vacation for two years and you want to communicate clearly that you understand this! Living on a Caribbean island presents many challenges, such as dealing with limited food/shopping supplies, power outages, extreme heat and weather, and distance from family and friends. While you will be able to have beach days for relaxation, living on a Caribbean island is not without some stress and you want to make sure your interviewer knows you understand that.

HOW WILL YOU COPE WITH BEING SO FAR AWAY FROM YOUR FAMILY?

The obvious answers are that you can Skype and FaceTime and see your family on vacations, assuming you can afford to fly home!

At least one major Caribbean medical school asks applicants to write a short essay during the interview, but this is reputed to be a low stress, easy exercise that evaluates your ability to communicate.

CHAPTER 17

THE SAMPLE INTERVIEW

Create an outline for your answers to the following questions, which are certainly going to be asked at most, if not all, of your interviews:

TELL ME ABOUT YOURSELF

This is what I call a launching pad question, which can come in other versions, such as "What brings you here today?" or "Tell me why you are here." This question presents an opportunity to paint a picture of yourself and present all of the information you hope to discuss in your interview. While you don't want to go into too much detail about any one activity or experience in your response, you do want to give your interviewer enough material so she can ask more questions about the topics you mention. Questions like this one are ice breakers and give you the opportunity to really control an interview and set the stage for what will be discussed. There are several ways to respond to this question, and I advise you to have a general outline (never memorize responses) of how you might answer it.

1. The chronological approach. This is the most common way to respond to this question. Interviewers want to know about your background, where you grew up, where you were educated, what is important to you both personally and academically. They want to understand what motivates and interests you. Provide a brief autobiographical statement that will provide the interviewer with tons of interesting aspects of who you are from which he or she can draw other questions.

2. The interests-based approach. Another way to answer this question is to outline your interests that make you who you are. In doing this, you can also describe when each of your curiosities started, how you pursued them and why they are each important to you.

3. A qualities or characteristics-based approach. Some applicants prefer to describe themselves in terms of who they are: I am loyal, curious, athletic, and interested in other populations. For each "quality" the student can discuss experiences that illustrate that quality.

Regardless of the approach, you should discuss both your personal, scholarly, and extracurricular background to offer a comprehensive response.

A SAMPLE ANSWER:

I am 26 years old and currently am working in oncology research. I grew up in Southern California with my parents, who emigrated from Russia. My grandparents also lived with us and we had a tightly knit family. I have been interested in medicine since my grandfather became sick when I was a freshman in high school. I had just started high school biology, and I often went with him to his doctor's appointments and helped him at home. I became curious about the drugs he was taking and what was going on with his body. I also was concerned about his emotional state and appreciated the vital role his doctor played in helping him cope with his illness. I have been volunteering in hospitals since that time. During high school I was also on the debate team and played varsity tennis. I enrolled in college and had a tough time my freshman year since I was not prepared for the more rigorous academic environment. But I improved my study skills and did better in subsequent years. I majored in biology with a minor in anthropology. I also gained extensive exposure to a variety of specialties through shadowing. After my junior year of college, I started working in the lab where I now work during the summer, and I have enjoyed my research so much that I decided to take this year to dedicate myself to it. Throughout college I also volunteered at a middle school tutoring underserved children and was heavily involved in the student government. Through my involvement in a nearby free clinic where I still volunteer I also gained a greater understanding of the challenges facing many US citizens. I have been looking forward to this day for a long time, and I was hoping to get an interview here and I thank you for inviting me.

WHY THIS IS A GOOD ANSWER:

The applicant creates a clear picture of himself, his motivations, and his path, along with his low grades his freshman year – a possible "red flag." Now his interviewer can "cherry pick" what he would like to discuss, including:

- His background
- What most impacted the applicant about his grandfather's care
- His research experience
- His low grades freshman year
- His shadowing experiences
- His tutoring experiences
- His academics
- His involvement in student government
- His involvement in a free clinic

WHY DO YOU WANT TO BE A DOCTOR?

You will undoubtedly be asked this question many times during your medical school interviews. When preparing for your medical school interviews, it is vital that you really think about what motivated you to pursue a career in medicine. A response such as, "I have always loved science and helping people," for example, won't cut it. I am always a bit surprised when I ask this question, and the student fails to mention anything about patient care. Be sure to mention helping patients as the cornerstone of your motivations to pursue a career in medicine. I encourage most clients to answer this question both in terms of "when" and "why." This enables you to tell the interviewer about your longstanding (ideally) motivation to pursue a career in medicine. You can also use segues to bring up various medically related experiences and your future career plans, which will provide your interviewer with more material to ask about. Offering a truly comprehensive response to this question, or any of its variants (When did you know you wanted to be a doctor? How do you know you want to be a doctor?) shows that you have made this decision over the long term and not on a whim. Remember that a career in medicine involves a love of learning, teaching (patients and possibly future students and residents), working with different populations, sometimes research, and service. Use your experiences to offer evidence for why you want to be a physician.

SAMPLE ANSWER:

Well, as I mentioned when we started talking, my interest in medicine really began when my grandfather was sick. He had heart disease and I was so intrigued by what was going on with his body and how his medications helped treat his illnesses. I was also inspired by the doctors who treated him and in particular by his cardiologist who was compassionate and really seemed to care about my grandfather and our family. Not only was this doctor technically competent and knowledgeable, but he also treated my grandfather as he would treat his own father. I could see that many physicians treated my grandfather differently because he was an immigrant and did not speak English well. But his cardiologist didn't do this, and I was determined to be like him – able to care for patients sensitively while being intellectually challenged and utilizing technical skills. Since then I have learned about research, and I now understand that in medicine I can combine a career in clinical medicine and research, which is what I hope to do in the future. I also hope to volunteer as a physician, probably domestically, because my work at the free clinic has shown me a need to help those who do not have access to care. I want to be a doctor to make a valuable contribution to people's health and well-being while making a more far-reaching impact through research.

WHY THIS IS A GOOD ANSWER:

- Student provides background to demonstrate the duration of his interest
- He demonstrates compassion, empathy and cultural
- competence
- He shows that he understands what it means to practice medicine
- He implies that he is intellectually curious
- He gives an idea of his future plans, which incorporate all of his past experiences and thus he seems directed and committed to a career in medicine
- He demonstrates his understanding of others and issues related to our health system by mentioning his free clinic work
- He provides segues and prompts for the interviewer
- to ask more questions

WHY OUR SCHOOL?

Medical schools are looking for the best candidates, but they are also seeking students who are the best fit for their school. It is essential that you research the school where you are interviewing and have specific reasons why you want to attend. Avoid "telling them what they want to hear" and choose things that are aligned with your demonstrated interests. For example, if you are an avid researcher with five original publications, do not be offended if a school focusing on primary care does not offer you an acceptance even if their average "stats" are lower than yours. You must convince the interviewer that you would be a good fit for the school and that you can best achieve your goals and ideals at that specific school.

SAMPLE ANSWER:

I want to go to your medical school for many reasons. First of all, the school has early clinical exposure, which I think is important and fosters an environment of collaboration through the use of small groups and problem based learning. I also appreciate the school's curriculum and the block system. I value that the student and patient populations are diverse, which is also important to me. I enjoy working with people who are different than I and learning about them, which is one of the reasons I enjoyed tutoring underserved children. If I were to become a student here I would do research, and the school is a leader in my field of research. I think that I would find many role models here who could help mentor me to become a physician scientist, and the educational environment would be stimulating. I am also interested in learning more about the impact of culture on how people perceive health care and there is an elective focused specifically on this topic, which I would pursue. And, I would join the student run clinic because this is work that I currently value now at the free clinic where I volunteer. I would also be thrilled to move to this city and experience a new part of the country.

WHY THIS IS A GOOD ANSWER:

Student shows he is knowledgeable and informed about the school

He identifies specific reasons why he is interested in the school

He presents himself as an ideal fit for the school by identifying some of his own values that mirror the school's philosophy and mission.

He mentions his own interest in research, which likely distinguishes him from other applicants and how he envisions making a contribution to the school.

He also mentions his tutoring and free clinic work, providing a prompt for his interviewer

CHAPTER 18

OTHER POPULAR QUESTIONS

TELL ME ABOUT A CHALLENGING TIME IN YOUR LIFE.

This is a very popular behavioral interview question. The interviewer may ask about a time when you weren't successful or about your greatest failure. "I can't think of anything" is the wrong answer. This response demonstrates lack of insight; we have all had challenges. The interviewer wants to know that you can cope with adversity and how you do it and that you learn from challenging times. He also wants to know that you are resilient and resourceful.

SAMPLE ANSWER:

A challenging time for me was when I started college. I had always done very well in high school, and I didn't expect that I would find college so difficult both academically and socially. It was the first time I lived away from my family, and I was homesick. I also found the work load heavier than in high school, and good grades did not come as easily. I learned to manage my time better and improved my study habits. But I also made a real effort to make new friends and adapt to my new environment. In retrospect, I realize that stepping out of my comfort zone was one of the best choices I ever made. This forced me to grow, mature, and adapt, and the skills I gained will help me in the future. I now understand that challenging myself helps me to grow in many ways.

WHY THIS IS A GOOD ANSWER:

- The student is honest and authentic
- He presents the challenge and the solutions
- He conveys that he can persevere
- He conveys that he learned from this experience
- He makes it clear that he understands that such situations are likely to occur again and that he is better equipped to cope with them

WHAT WOULD YOU SAY IS ONE OF THE MAJOR PROBLEMS WITH OUR HEALTH CARE SYSTEM TODAY?

As I have mentioned, no one expects you to be an expert in health policy. If asked this question (and many interviewers don't even touch on this topic because it is so complex), you want to convey that you have an overall understanding of the issues and that you realize that they are complicated. I suggest that applicants read about health care reform during their application year at least once a week so they feel better prepared to discuss these issues, but my impression is that few interviewees are asked in detail about health care reform.

SAMPLE ANSWER:

Wow. The issues of health care reform are so complex, and I am trying to grasp them. I think one of the biggest concerns is lack of access to care for the uninsured. For example, at the free clinic where I work, many patients present with complications of disease and we must then refer them to the emergency department for further care. This is because they do not have access to primary providers and because they often do not take their medications or care for themselves. I think if we increased awareness of prevention for underserved communities and made it easier somehow for them to live healthier lifestyles and increased their access to care by providing them with some kind of coverage, we would decrease our health care spending because these actions would help prevent disease.

WHY THIS IS A GOOD ANSWER:

- The interviewee admits he has a lot to learn
- He then goes on to explain some of the issues with access to care, patient education, and patient compliance
- He also demonstrates cultural competence by recognizing that achieving a healthy lifestyle is not easy for certain populations
- He suggests some solutions to these problems
- He mentions his firsthand experience caring for the underserved

DO YOU HAVE ANY QUESTIONS FOR ME?

Most students feel they must have questions to ask at the close of an interview, but unless you have an interviewer whom you sense wants you to ask a question, it is not always necessary to do so. Realize that not everyone agrees with me on this point, and some people advise applicants always to ask questions, regardless of the circumstances. But I feel this is disingenuous, and I could always tell when applicants asked questions because they thought it was the right thing to do. Not only was this a waste of time for both of us, but it sometimes diluted positive feelings I had about the interview before then.

The applicant must also pay attention to an interviewer's cues, however. For example, if an interviewer says, "So, what questions do you have for me?" it implies that you should have some. (If your interviewer is an Egomaniac or a "talker," he likely will want you to ask questions.) But if she asks, "Do you have any questions?" coming up with something is not obligatory. A good strategy is to ask questions during your interview, assuming it has a conversational tone. This has the advantage of seeming more natural and sincere and allows you, when asked about any additional queries at the end of the interview, to answer truthfully, "You have already answered all my questions."

If you feel you must ask questions or you are most comfortable having questions (I find this is the case for many applicants), you should try to ask questions that relate to your interests and demonstrate your interest in and knowledge of the school. It is also safe to ask about how much elective time students receive to pursue their interests in other specialties, if the school has a formal mentorship program, if students receive guidance when it is time to apply to residency or, if you have a specific interest, you can ask about opportunities in that area. Don't ask questions that you could easily find out the answers to on the school's website.

I advise students to ask questions about something they learned about during interview day. Depending on the structure of your interview, you likely had tours and introductory meetings where you have learned about the medical school. Draw from this information; it shows you are paying attention and that your questions aren't scripted. It is better to ask questions about specific opportunities, aspects of the curriculum, and rotations. Stay away from questions that start with "why" since they can come off sounding critical. For example, "Why are students required to complete a thesis?" Instead, try this: "I am really intrigued by the thesis requirement since I already have an interest in public health that I would hope to pursue as a student here. In the past, have students done thesis work in public health and could I start exploring that interest earlier than my senior year?"

SAMPLE ANSWER #1:

I don't have any specific questions. I have studied every page of the school's website because I am so interested in this school. The presentation and tour today were also very thorough, so I feel that all of my questions have been answered. I would be really happy to attend medical school here and think it would be a great fit for me. The school's commitment to underserved populations, the opportunities for early clinical work in the student run clinic, as well as the global health programs all appeal to me. I also appreciate the flexibility I'd have as a fourth year student to do electives in what interests me. I was also hoping to move to the city for medical school because it's close to my family whom I have missed while in school in Chicago. If I think of any additional questions after I leave, to whom should I address these? Thanks for everything.

WHY THIS IS A GOOD ANSWER:

- It communicates to the interviewer that he prepared for the interview
- It communicates to the interviewer that he is informed about the school
- It demonstrates honesty and authenticity
- It transforms the question into a statement about his enthusiasm for the school
- By making this transformation the interviewer forgets what he asked the applicant in the first place
- It expresses gratitude for being considered and interviewed

SAMPLE ANSWER #2:

Most of my questions have been addressed today, and I must say that I think this school is the perfect fit for me. But, I was wondering how many students actually work at the student run free clinic and if there might be opportunities for me to take on a significant role there since I am interested in working with such populations not only in medical school but in my future career.

WHY THIS IS A GOOD ANSWER:

- The student communicates that he is prepared
- The student expresses his interest in the school
- The student asks about something that is related to his interest.
- The student demonstrates that he plans on taking on a significant role outside of the classroom while a medical student.

WHAT IS YOUR GREATEST WEAKNESS OR GREATEST STRENGTH?

Personally, I can't stand these questions and never asked them. Every medical school applicant has a prepared response for these questions which I find to be disingenuous and tells me little about him or her. I find that it is typically the unskilled interviewer who poses this question, but medical school applicants are always nervous about fielding these questions. Most often, applicants are advised to choose a strength that is actually a weakness, such as "I am a perfectionist." "I have a tough time saying no to opportunities." "I sometimes work so hard that I sacrifice my free time." I suggest simply being sincere. Give a real, honest answer but not one that would be a deal breaker for medical school, such as "I can't work on teams."

SAMPLE ANSWER:

I tend to procrastinate. I am constantly trying to improve this weakness because my procrastination causes me a lot of stress. And, when I get stressed because I am close to a deadline or exam, I am not very pleasant to be around. But, this stress is also what motivates me to get the job done.

WHY THIS IS A GOOD ANSWER:

- This applicant cites a real weakness
- He gives it a positive "spin"
- He appears authentic and genuine

A 16-year-old girl comes to your office with her mother. As you do routinely, you ask the mother to leave so you can talk to the girl openly. The patient confides in you that she is sexually active and asks you to prescribe birth control pills, but she does not want her mother to know. What do you do?

Ethical and "behavioral" questions can be tough. The "right" answers are not always obvious, and the key is to consider all aspects of the described situation and to consider what is in the best interest of the patient. The interviewer is looking for your "answer," of course, but he is also interested in your thought process, reasoning, ability to verbalize and to identify the issues and be sensitive to them, and whether you communicate that you are compassionate and considerate. Typically these types of questions are also designed to evaluate your professionalism, ability to work as a member of a team, values, ethics, and cultural competence.

SAMPLE ANSWER:

This is a tough question. First of all, I would educate the patient about the risk of unprotected sex with regard to sexually transmitted diseases and HIV. I would let her know that pregnancy was not the only consideration. I would also make sure she was sexually active because she wanted to be and that she was in no way being pressured. I would then ask what she was using for birth control. I would tell her that her mother should be aware that she is sexually active and of the risks of taking birth control pills and strongly advise her to take her mother into her confidence. However, I would offer this advice within the context of an assessment of the relationship she has with her mother. Ultimately, I don't know if I would prescribe the pills because it would depend on that state's laws regarding treating a minor, but I would want to protect this girl and wouldn't want her to become pregnant because I didn't prescribe her the medication. At the same time, I wouldn't want to encourage her sexual activity by giving her the prescription. I think I would seek out help from a social worker and would make sure to schedule a follow-up appointment with this patient once I had time to consider the legal issues and to learn more about other issues in her life and her family situation.

WHY THIS IS A GOOD ANSWER:

- The applicant considers this situation from multiple perspectives
- He considers how his actions will impact not only the patient but her family and the individual with whom she is having a sexual relationship
- He demonstrates that he thinks clearly and objectively
- He admits that he doesn't know the applicable laws
- but is aware that they vary by state
- He demonstrates compassion, empathy, professionalism,

and an understanding of the complexities of the situation
- He demonstrates resourcefulness and his ability to consider the other members of his "team"

WHY ARE YOU INTERESTED IN OUR MEDICAL SCHOOL?

In reality, we find that many interviewers do not ask this question. But, it is good to prepare for this question so you know as much about the medical school as possible before interview day. As I have mentioned elsewhere in this book, it is ideal if you can add information about why you are interested in the specific medical school at which you are interviewing during regular conversation, but this isn't always possible or natural. The key thing to address if you are asked "why our medical school?" is that you have done your research, know about what the school can offer you and what you can offer the school. In asking this question, your interviewer wants to know that you will be a productive member of the medical school community. Things to know about the medical school before you interview:

1. What is the school's mission?
2. What is the school's curriculum and what stands out about that curriculum?
3. Where is the school located and what are the demographics of that area?
4. Where are the school's affiliate locations where you are likely to do rotations and what are the demographics of those areas?
5. What extracurricular opportunities are of interest? What about clubs?

6. Are there any research opportunities that interest you?
7. Any programs in public or global health that interest you?
8. What is the general culture of the school and the student body?

SAMPLE ANSWER:

There are so many reasons I am particularly interested in Master Medical School. First of all, the location really appeals to me. I want to go to medical school in an urban setting where I will learn about the challenges facing underserved populations. My goal is to some day have a private practice along with an academic practice in a school just like this. I also love this city and with the limited free time I have, I will have plenty of things to do with my classmates. I also felt during today that I really fit in with the students I met. They are all so interesting, smart, and friendly. The early exposure to clinical medicine and the flexibility students have during their medical school years are also intriguing. I have many established interests as you can see, but I also hope to learn about other specialties in medicine and explore different areas of research. The cardiology research I did as an undergraduate fascinated me and I met one student who spent her summer after first year of medical school doing research with a leader in the field. That is really exciting to me. As a side note, I love to sing and the student a cappella group would be really great to be a part. Overall, I am think this school is a great fit for me and I would be a great fit for the school!

WHY THIS IS A GOOD ANSWER:

- The student is enthusiastic about the medical school. Positive and enthusiastic energy will bolster a response of this type.
- The student mentions the curriculum.
- The student mentions rotations - many applicants fail to think about their education beyond the first two years!
- The student discusses the location.
- The student makes it clear that she connected with current students, which shows she is collaborative and friendly.

WHERE DO YOU SEE YOURSELF IN THE FUTURE?

When answering this question or a question that asks about future goals, you must realize that you do not need to know what specialty you will pursue when answering this question! Rather, it is important to think globally about what qualities you hope to posses, the role you hope to play in patients' lives, as well as the role you will play in the medical and surrounding communities.

SAMPLE ANSWER:

I have shadowed several different types of physicians and I can see aspects of each specialty that I might enjoy. Therefore, I am not sure yet what specialty I might be interested in for residency. However, regardless of the specialty I pursue, I plan to offer the best care I can to my patients treating each of them as an individual. I understand the importance of practicing evidenced-based medicine so I hope to keep up to date with the advances in my specialty and to never stop learning. I might want to pursue a career in academic medicine because I enjoy teaching. Finally, I hope to be involved in my local community so I can impact others even when I am not in the hospital or office. I also plan to be involved in my local medical community so I am respected by my colleagues and that we all work together.

WHY THIS IS A GOOD ANSWER:

- The applicant makes it clear that she is curious and is honest that she isn't sure what specialty she's pursuing.
- She is going to put "patient care" first!
- She plans to be a lifelong learner and teacher.
- She understands her role in the local and medical communities.

CHAPTER 19

OTHER TOPICS AND QUESTIONS
YOU MAY BE ASKED

I do not pose answers to the following potpourri of questions or topics you may be asked to address because I strongly discourage applicants from simply telling interviewers what they think they want to hear. How you deal with the following will depend on your background and experiences; demonstrating authenticity, honesty, and consistency is key, so should any of these questions or subjects come up, address them in a fashion that is consistent with your application, experience, and letters of reference.

If you had a free day what would you do?

How do you achieve balance in your life?

Tell me a joke.

Teach me something.

What experience(s) made you want to pursue medicine?

How would your best friend describe you? What would he or she say is your greatest weakness?

What activity have you pursued on your own without the

influence of your parents?

What is something you tried really hard at but didn't turn out as expected or what has been your greatest challenge?

Did you ever have to work to help support yourself or fund your education?

How do you remember everything you have to do? How will you deal with debt?
Where have you traveled around the world?

Would you change anything in your background? What and why?

What would you do if you could not pursue a career in medicine?

Tell me about your research/volunteer/clinical/global health/public health/teaching experiences.

Explain your academic path.

What strengths would you bring to the medical school?

Why did you do a special master's program/MBA etc.?

Explain your poor grade/MCAT/academic performance.

How would you add to the diversity of our school?
Tell me about an ethical dilemma and how you decided

what to do.

What qualities should a physician possess?

What qualities do you possess that will help you to become a physician?

Tell me about the most influential person in your life.

Tell me about your most valued mentor. What is your most valuable accomplishment? What direct clinical exposure do you have?

What leadership roles have you held? Why should we choose you?

What should I tell the admissions committee about you?

Describe your perfect day.

Where do you see yourself in the future (10, 20, or 30 years)?

If you could change anything about your education, what would that be and why?

What kinds of books do you read? Tell me about the book you read most recently.

How do you feel about medical students not being allowed

to have cell phones in the hospital?

What do you do for fun?

In closing, is there anything else you would like to tell me?

What have you done since you graduated from college?

CHAPTER 20
QUESTIONS TO ASK YOUR INTERVIEWER

The best questions to ask interviewers relate to your own interests and background. Ideally, the questions you ask should be "organic" and based on actual questions you come up with during the day based on what you learn about the medical school. Below are some basic questions you can ask your faculty interviewer.

GENERAL:

How would you describe a typical medical student here? What are the most positive aspects of this school?

How do you like being on faculty here? What do you do/what is your specialty?

CURRICULUM:

Do you anticipate any upcoming changes to the curriculum? Can I access lectures via the web or on line?

Do students typically do research for credit?

What do most students do during their first year summer? Are there global health opportunities?

What are the options for fourth year elective rotations?

MENTORING:

Is there a formal guidance program here?

Do students receive help when applying for residency?

Are clinical faculty supportive of students?

ROTATIONS:

Do students have bedside teaching on rotations?

Are rotations crowded; do students compete for patients, procedures, or teaching?

Where do students complete most clinical rotations?

AFTER MEDICAL SCHOOL:

What are the most popular specialties that students pursue?

What percentage of students complete residencies at hospitals affiliated with the medical school?

PART 3:

THE MULTIPLE MINI INTERVIEW

CHAPTER 21

WHAT IS THE MULTIPLE MINI INTERVIEW (MMI)?

The Multiple Mini Interview, initially developed by McMaster University School of Medicine in Canada, is a station-based interview used to assess an applicant's "soft skills," qualities, characteristics, values, ideals, and decision making skills. Studies have shown that the MMI decreases interviewer and evaluation bias and can better predict a future medical student's performance, professionalism, and performance on clinical tests than the traditional interview. These data, together with a move towards holistic admissions in the United States, have resulted in more and more medical schools' favoring this interview style over the traditional one- on- one interview. We anticipate that every year more medical schools will replace traditional interview formats with the MMI.

A typical MMI interview consists of a circuit of eight to 10 stations through which interviewees rotate. All stations are usually in a single hallway, making it easy for applicants to move from station to station. Often referred to as the "speed dating' interview, the MMI presents a new scenario, task, or situation and a new evaluator at each station. The circuit also includes rest stations (usually two), which offer the opportunity to use a bathroom. Interviewees are allowed a total of 10 minutes at each station before they have to move on to the next.. The interviewee spends the first two minutes outside the room at each station reviewing the scenario, question, or task that he or she will have to talk about or complete in the room. The next eight minutes are then spent in the room discussing the scenario, role playing, or completing the required task.

Keep in mind, however, that the exact set up of an MMI will vary from one institution to another. Some medical schools may have only six stations whereas others have hybrid interviews, which are a combination of the MMI and a traditional interview.

Here is the standard set up and sequence for each MMI station:

Bell rings indicating the start of the next station.

Applicant takes a clipboard posted outside the station or posted on the station door and has two minutes to read the scenario, role, question, or task. The instructions are often slightly vague, which is deliberate.

Bell rings indicating the interviewee can enter the room, where another copy of the scenario or task is available for reference..

Applicant has eight minutes to discuss the scenario, role play, complete the required task, or answer the posted question.

Bell rings indicating the end of the session and applicant exits the room. Feedback is never provided in the room.

Applicant proceeds to next station and the cycle starts again.

Evaluator rates applicant after he or she exits.

The entire MMI circuit lasts anywhere from 70 - 100 minutes depending on the institution.

Here is a typical roster of the type of subjects you can expect to address at various stations on an MMI interview day:

- Professionalism
- Dealing with stress
- Problem solving
- Interpersonal skills
- Culture/diversity
- Ethics (two stations)
- Pathway to medicine (traditional medical school interview question)
- Teamwork - giving instructions to a partner
- Teamwork - receiving instructions from a partner

Applicants are usually, but not always, allowed to jot down notes during this process but typically have time for that only during the two minute period before entering the room.

WHO ARE YOUR MMI RATERS AND EVALUATORS?

In the MMI, your evaluators are referred to as "raters" and not as "interviewers." As you can imagine, the MMI requires a tremendous workforce of raters. While most medical schools recruit their own faculty and administrators to serve as raters, some schools also recruit and train civilians from outside of the medical community for these roles. Therefore, it is good to know that the people evaluating you will be a diverse group with regard to background, profession, and perspective. Sometimes schools also allow alumni, students, or residents to participate. Usually you will not be told who your evaluators are - either before or after your interview day.

All raters will be trained on how to evaluate you. They may also be given additional information or have knowledge of a scenario or policy that you do not have. Don't let this intimidate you. Raters are instructed to "follow the interviewees' lead" and not to direct them. Scenarios and questions are typically open-ended and somewhat vague, which allows the interviewee to offer original approaches to the scenario. The rater will not guide the applicant but might challenge her.

CHAPTER 22
MMI STATION TYPES

SCENARIO-BASED DISCUSSION

A scenario- based discussion is the most typical type of MMI station, usually ethical in nature, and can involve every day scenarios, those that take place in a medical setting, or real-life medical or policy scenarios that present an ethical dilemma. In this type of scenario, the rater will usually have follow up questions for the interviewee. These questions will be individually tailored and based on each interviewee's approach to the scenario.

ROLE PLAY

At these stations raters will inform the interviewee about his or her role in the scenario before the session begins. An actor who will play another "role" in the scenario also will be present, along with an evaluator. These stations typically involve an "uncomfortable" confrontation with the actor that might relate to giving bad news or asking why the actor hasn't followed through on something or was dishonest in some way. The interviewee, who plays the role of the interviewer in the scenario, speaks with and engages the actor as if in a real life encounter. The rater grades the interviewer on this interaction.

TEAMWORK OR TASK STATION

Working as a member of a team is vital in medicine so teamwork stations are pretty common on MMI interviews. Teamwork stations usually involve two applicants working together on a task. Usually students must have their backs to each other so communication is only verbal. You will typically have two teamwork or task stations on interview day. At one teamwork station you will be asked to be the "giver" and will give direction for a complex task to another applicant. At another you might be asked to be the "receiver" and take direction from a fellow applicant. This station usually has two raters - one is assigned to each interviewee. In teamwork exercises, when you are asked to complete a task, typically with another student, effective communication skills are imperative. You will be evaluated by your ability to work with someone else, to listen, and to communicate effectively. Most of the tasks are complex, or even impossible, so you must not lose patience or get frustrated when you are on either "end" of this task. Tasks usually involve drawing, completing a puzzle, building Legos or another type of structural element, or doing origami.

STANDARD INTERVIEW QUESTIONS

Many MMI interviews have "standard question" stations where applicants are asked common interview questions such as:

• Why do you want to be a doctor?
• Why are you interested in our school?

- Tell me about yourself.
- Where do you see yourself in the future?.
- Tell me about your path to medicine.

CHAPTER 23

WHAT DOES THE MMI ASSESS?

In an MMI, raters will evaluate you on the following:

1) COMMUNICATION SKILLS

Whether you are participating in a scenario, role playing, or doing a teamwork exercise, the entire MMI process requires excellent communication skills. In acting stations, you may well find yourself counseling the actor since these stations often involve a problem that you try to solve. You will be evaluated on your ability to communicate well, show empathy, really listen, and connect with and engage others. Any hint of being condescending, opinionated, self-righteous, bossy, or closed-minded will not go over well with your rater!

2) CRITICAL THINKING

Your ability to critically evaluate a scenario, identify what additional information could help you reach a resolution, and knowing what questions to ask are vital. (Look for more about critical thinking later in this book.)

3) ETHICS

Having a fundamental understanding of ethical principles, also described in more detail later in the book, will help you navigate ethical and policy based scenarios intelligently and thoughtfully.

4) CULTURAL COMPETENCE AND UNDERSTANDING

Inevitably, at least one of your scenarios will put you in a position to demonstrate cultural competence and your understanding of people who have backgrounds and cultural norms that are different from your own. Acknowledging any distinctive cultural norms when discussing a scenario will show your cultural competence.

5) PROFESSIONALISM

Some scenarios are meant to make it a bit difficult for you to demonstrate patience, understanding of others' limitations and weaknesses, or to maintain your cool without getting emotional or saying anything inconsiderate. Maintaining a professional demeanor throughout the entire MMI interview is key to success.

6) INTERPERSONAL SKILLS

Throughout the MMI you are being evaluated on how well you communicate, both verbally and via body language, along with your overall demeanor and how you treat others. Raters want to see your skill in connecting with people and how quickly you understand the emotional tenor of a scenario or situation. This is why extroverts and people who naturally enjoy engaging and learning about others do so well in this process.

7) TEAMWORK /ABILITY TO COLLABORATE

How you would interact with others, both in terms of offering direction, as well as listening and taking direction, are assessed in task stations. Since you will be working with others as a member of a team throughout your medical education and career, being tolerant of others and working through collaborative challenges are important.

8) PROBLEM SOLVING SKILLS

How you solve problems, and how knowledgeable you are about what you need to solve problems, will be considered in numerous stations. Problems solving skills are linked closely with critical thinking skills; you must be able to identify what other information might be helpful to navigate a particular scenario.

9) CONFIDENCE

While your rater is not actually looking for confidence in applicants, I have included this quality here because interviewees who display confidence naturally do better during the MMI process and are perceived in a better light by everyone around them. You will be nervous on your interview day, and that is expected, but if you are prepared and know what is in store that nervousness will subside, leaving you confident and able to think on your feet.

10) COMPASSION, THOUGHTFULNESS, AND EMPATHY

Raters want to know that you can put yourself in another person's shoes, understand his or her situation and perspective, and be able to relate and connect to another human being in a thoughtful and considerate way. They want to see your ability to connect to another person. Such qualities are more easily evaluated through a scenario-based format such as the MMI.

You will read more about each of these crucial elements throughout the book.

YOUR VOICE, DEMEANOR, AND EXPRESSION AND THE MMI

When you meet someone, think of what makes them approachable and likable. Do the following come to mind?

- Has a smile
- Speaks clearly (not too fast or too slow) and at a normal volume (not too loud or soft)
- Carries himself with confidence and has good posture
- Is approachable and looks me in the eye
- Appears open and receptive by leaning in slightly on his chair, rather than slouching, and nods to show she's listening
- Seems interested in meeting me
- Is attentive and not distracted
- Acts self-assured and confident (but not arrogant or over-confident)

When you enter the MMI room, the rater will immediately get an impression of you based on these factors. So look the interviewer in the eye. Say "hello." Walk with confidence and good posture. Smile. Then jump into the discussion or scenario or task. By the same token, if someone else is in the room, such as another student in a task station or an actor, be open and approachable with them, too. Even though the MMI interview is designed to minimize subjective evaluations and bias, they inevitably exist.

CHAPTER 24

ETHICAL AND POLICY
SCENARIOS OR QUESTIONS

The key to success in an MMI interview is to think quickly and communicate your thoughts succinctly, clearly, and logically. Raters are also assessing a student's ability to consider all aspects of a problem or situation so becoming adept at this is key. To illustrate your ability to think critically, you must also know what information you don't have or you could use to make a more informed decision.

Since some stations involve current issues or polices in medicine, it is smart to read about policy issues in healthcare. This is not because you need to have knowledge for the MMI interview but because understanding the current climate in medicine will improve your ability to think critically about challenging policies. We recommend periodic review of the Kaiser website for this purpose: https://www.kff.org

We advise students to practice their ethical decision making skills while preparing for the MMI. When faced with an ethical dilemma or situation, you must demonstrate your ability to think and consider all aspects of the situation as well as the ramifications of all possible decisions. It is also essential to consider the perspective of each "stakeholder" in a scenario, whether a patient, a husband or sister, a nurse, a hospital, or another entity that's involved. By doing so, you will demonstrate your thoughtfulness, empathy, and maturity.

BIOETHICAL PRINCIPLES AND ETHICAL DECISION MAKING

Understanding bioethical principles and some basics about ethical decision making will also help students prepare for the ethically based scenarios in the MMI. Below are five common ethical principles that come into play when discussing ethical scenarios during the MMI. You don't need to use the "labels" we have given these elements during the interview, but having a basic understanding of them during a discussion of an ethical scenario will allow you to better navigate that scenario and not miss any crucial considerations.

1) TRUTHFULNESS AND CONFIDENTIALITY

Truthfulness means telling the truth to someone who has the right to know even if that truth is painful. By the same token, it is a doctor's obligation to keep information confidential. For example, if a patient is diagnosed with terminal cancer, truthfulness dictates that the doctor must tell the patient about the diagnosis even though this will be difficult news to hear. However, if the patient asks the doctor not to disclose this information to the patient's spouse, the doctor is ethically obligated to keep this information confidential.

2) AUTONOMY

Autonomy refers to each person's right to make his or her own choices, including those related to medical care. This means she can refuse necessary treatment or disregard a doctor's instructions. You will often be faced with scenarios in which a patient wants to refuse treatment or not do what the doctor feels is best.

3) INFORMED CONSENT

This refers to the patient's right to understand the risks and benefits of any medical procedure he is about to undergo. This also means the patient must understand what might happen if the procedure is not carried out.

4) BENEFICENCE AND NONMALEFICENCE

Beneficence means "doing good" or doing what is in the patient's best interests whereas nonmaleficence means to "do no harm" or avoiding harm. In all scenarios, you must do good and make decisions that are in the best interest of anyone involved in the scenario. Likewise, you must not make any decisions that might result in harm to any of the stakeholders in the scenario.

5) JUSTICE

It is important to be fair to all people. This seems obvious but, in all scenarios, always consider every element of the situation and how you can be most fair to all of the stakeholders

CRITICAL THINKING SKILLS

The MMI also evaluates critical thinking skills, which typically come into play in scenarios that involve ethical issues in policy and healthcare. The Kaiser Family Foundation has an excellent website that discusses current policy issues. I advise students to review this material periodically during the interview season: https://www.kff.org. By familiarizing yourself with the issues you will develop an understanding of the ethical challenges involved in many policies, which will offer you a comfortable foundation for the MMI. No one expects you to be a policy expert, however, so don't be alarmed if you encounter an unfamiliar policy or issue at your interview.

The MMI is not testing your knowledge. What is crucial is how you use your previous knowledge and experiences to reason through the scenario with the information you already have. As I have mentioned, demonstrating that you understand all sides of a situation and can consider the viewpoints and consequences for all stakeholders in a scenario are key. Raters want to see that you can reason through issues relevant to society.

Also imperative is to understand that there is never a "right answer" for ethical scenarios. And rarely is there a "perfect" resolution, and expressing that is fine as long as you demonstrate how you've come to that conclusion. What raters want to see is that you can adopt a stance, defend that stance, and discuss issues related to it. Your rater may have knowledge that you do not, which enables him to challenge you a bit. What is key is to stay strong and not to waver.

TALKING ABOUT YOUR OWN EXPERIENCES

While it isn't always possible, talking about your own life experiences and how they might relate to a prompt can serve multiple purposes. First of all, this gives you the chance to talk about yourself and offer more information about your attributes and suitability for a career in medicine. It also helps to explain your thought process, how you came to your conclusions about a given scenario, and how you think. At most MMI interviews raters will encourage you to infuse your own experiences when discussing a scenario or in an acting station. However, keep in mind that you should talk about your life experiences only when it is appropriate.

So - what is the best way to approach an ethical or policy-based scenario?

After reading a scenario, think about it within this framework:

- Consider what facts and information you have
- Identify the key ethical issues
- Identify the parties or stakeholders involved
- Identify potential consequences
- Consider the ethical principles (autonomy, truthfulness, and confidentiality, beneficence, nonmaleficence, justice)
- Think about the possible actions and outsourcing/ consultations that might help you and the parties involved in the scenario
- Do you need more information? What don't you know that might help your decision or course of action?
- Discuss any life experiences that help you reach your

conclusions

- Be prepared to defend or justify your actions

Consider all of the scenarios offered in this book and practice, practice, practice!

CHAPTER 25

ROLE PLAY OR ACTING SCENARIO

Many applicants really enjoy the opportunity to role play, but others are not comfortable in this setting. If you have any acting experience, this kind of station should be easy! When you read an acting prompt, immediately do your best to "get in character." Assume the role you are assigned, start thinking like that person, and come up with what you will say first to the actor. The key to role playing scenarios is also to be flexible and to listen carefully. Engage the actor and be as open as possible so the actor is comfortable talking to you. Since this station is about dialogue, it is important to go with the flow in these scenarios. You really can't predict how the actor will respond to your initial statement or question in the room. Also offer your own life experiences to the actor when it's appropriate.

Typically you will be presented with a problem related to the actor and are asked to help the actor work through that problem. So, before you go in the room, consider what your stance will be. How do you hope to help the actor? What questions do you want to ask? Try to think of more than one solution to the "problem." Make suggestions and give options. Always serve as an advocate and ally for the actor in the room. Offer concrete ways to help.

HERE ARE SOME TYPICAL SCENARIOS:

- Talking to a member of your team or study group about how she is not participating
- Giving bad news
- Offering comfort to someone who is anxious or stressed
- Having to take responsibility for something you did that was wrong or a mistake that you made
- Confronting someone who did something unethical
- Talking to someone who might not be taking care of herself – engaging in drinking, drugs, risky behavior

Having a normal conversation is what works best. Some general rules to follow for this type of station are:

Start the session with an open ended question, such as "How are things going today? What have you been up to?"

Always show understanding and compassion for the actor's situation and circumstance.

Demonstrate that you are listening to what he or she is saying through your language, tone of voice, and gestures, such as by nodding, and "leaning in."

In these scenarios always show respect, kindness, consideration, and warmth toward the actor. You want to convey that you are a kind person who is open and receptive to others.

Never interrupt the actor when he or she is speaking.

In other words, in acting scenarios, be on your best behavior and treat others as you would want to be treated. Never be rude, curt, or judgmental and don't lecture!!! The idea here is to have open and considerate dialogue with the actor. Even if the actor loses patience or becomes frustrated, you must always maintain a calm and considerate demeanor.

CHAPTER 26
TASK OR COLLABORATION STATIONS

Approached the right way, task and collaboration stations can actually be quite fun. My primary advice is to stay calm, speak clearly, listen attentively, and don't get frustrated!!! Also be sure not to interrupt the person speaking. In these stations you also will be asked to be the "receiver" and complete a task based on directions given by another student. Or you will be asked to be the "giver" by offering guidance to another student who is completing a task.

The tasks offered are often quite complex or even impossible. This is not an accident. Raters want to know that you can communicate and listen effectively under duress and that you won't get frustrated or lose patience when things aren't going so smoothly or easily. Typical task stations involve drawing a picture, doing origami, or building something with Legos or another material. If you do feel frustrated, remember the scenario is only eight minutes and soon will be over. This is not a test of whether or not you can complete a task or instruct someone else to; it is a test of your patience, communication skills, and ability to work with others.

WHAT YOU SHOULD DO DEPENDS ON WHETHER YOU ARE A "GIVER" OR A "RECEIVER."

IF YOU ARE A GIVER:

Be clear and immediately tell the receiver what his or her task is: "Your job is to build an airplane out of the Legos in front of you, and I am going to explain how to do this as easily as I can."

Be open: "If you have any questions, please ask me."

Be encouraging: "I know it might be frustrating, but you are doing really well!"

Also ask for feedback: "Is there anything I can do to make the instructions clearer?"

Never judge through what you say, your body language, your expression, or your tone of voice.

Compliment the receiver. "You are a really great listener."

Don't interrupt the receiver.

IF YOU ARE A RECEIVER:

Be a good listener!

Express gratitude to the giver. "Thank you. Those instructions are really great."

If you need more direction and aren't sure what to do don't be afraid to ask politely for more instruction: "I think I understand what you are trying to say, but, I am not 100% sure. Could you please explain that last step again?"

Don't interrupt the giver.

If the giver seems stumped or frustrated, offer support: "This seems like a really tough task. I think you are doing a great job offering direction."

HOW APPLICANTS ARE RATED

Raters are asked to evaluate applicants based on:

Communication skills
Strengths of arguments displayed
Applicants' suitability for the medical profession

Applicants are evaluated on a scale of 1 to 10. One is considered "unsuitable" for a career in medicine and 10 is considered outstanding.

For each type of station, the rater will be asked to assign this 'grade' based on different criteria but, in the end, each rater grades each applicant on the 1 through 10 scale. Raters are asked to assign this numeric assessment based on the pool of applicants he or she is evaluating. In our experience, however, this does not mean students are rated on a "curve" and everyone in a single group of students can do well.

There is also a space for any comments the rater might have.

HOW TO PREPARE FOR THE MMI

PRACTICE UNDER TIMED CIRCUMSTANCES.

You will have two minutes to read and consider each scenario before going into the interview. Becoming adept at creating an outline in your mind and doing this efficiently will decrease nervousness and anxiety. When you read a scenario consider what information is MISSING or what other information could help you make an informed decision.

Because you have only eight minutes per station, you want to make sure you can communicate your points effectively. By the same token, you don't want to have too little to say! Understanding how long eight minutes "feels" when discussing a scenario will make you more comfortable on interview day. This means you should practice addressing scenario responses by timing yourself.

Practice multiple prompts on any given day. MMI interview days are tiring and, while adrenaline is likely to get you through a day even if you are tired, practicing a series of prompts will help you avoid fatigue at the MMI.

Read the Kaiser website so you are familiar with current issues in medicine: https://www.kff.org. Search the web for other useful sites. We also like the New York Times and Wall Street Journal health sections. The idea is not to attain knowledge, necessarily, but to gain an understanding of current issues and ethical dilemmas.

Practice role playing. It is actually fun once you get the hang of it!

MedEdits plans to add more and more MMI scenarios to our database so visit our website often for practice scenarios.

CHAPTER 27

MEDICAL SCHOOLS THAT USE THE MMI

This list includes medical schools that were using the MMI when this book was written. Keep in mind that more schools may have adopted this model since.

UNITED STATES ALLOPATHIC MEDICAL SCHOOLS:

- Albany Medical College
- California Northstate
- Central Michigan University
- Chicago Medical School at Rosalind Franklin University
- Cooper Medical School of Rowan University (hybrid—traditional + MMI)
- Duke University
- Michigan State University College of Human Medicine
- New York Medical College
- New York University
- Nova Southeastern (MD)
- Oregon Health and Science University
- Rutgers Robert Wood Johnson Medical School
- San Juan Bautista (Puerto Rico)
- Stanford University

- SUNY Upstate
- Tufts University (Maine Track only)
- Universidad Central Del Caribe (Puerto Rico)
- University of Alabama (hybrid)
- University of Arizona
- University of California-Davis
- University of California-Los Angeles
- University of California-Riverside
- University of California-San Diego
- University of Cincinnati
- University of Colorado
- University of Massachusetts
- University of Michigan (hybrid)
- University of Minnesota Twin Cities
- University of Mississippi
- University of Missouri-Kansas City
- University of Nevada
- University of South Carolina Greenville (hybrid)
- University of Texas–Austin
- University of Toledo
- University of Utah (hybrid)
- University of Vermont
- Virginia Commonwealth
- Virginia Tech Carilion
- Wake Forest
- Wayne State (hybrid)
- Western Michigan University (hybrid)

UNITED STATES OSTEOPATHIC MEDICAL SCHOOLS:

- AT Still University – School of Osteopathic Medicine in Arizona
- Marian University College of Osteopathic Medicine
- Michigan State College of Osteopathic Medicine
- Pacific Northwest College of Osteopathic Medicine
- University of North Texas
- University of the Incarnate Word School of Osteopathic Medicine
- Western University of Health Sciences College of Osteopathic Medicine (hybrid)

CANADIAN ALLOPATHIC MEDICAL SCHOOLS:

- Dalhousie University Faculty of Medicine
- Laval University Faculty of Medicine
- McGill University Faculty of Medicine
- McMasterUniversity, Michael G.DeGroote School of Medicine Northern Ontario School of Medicine
- Queen's University Faculty of Health Sciences
- Universite de Montreal Faculty of Medicine
- University of Alberta Faculty of Medicine and Dentistry
- University of British Columbia Faculty of Medicine
- University of Calgary Faculty of Medicine
- University of Manitoba Faculty of Medicine
- University of Saskatchewan College of Medicine
- University of Sherbrooke Faculty of Medicine

CHAPTER 28

MMI KEY TIPS AND REVIEW

1. With a station based format that moves quickly, it is important to leave each scenario or station in the room behind you when you move to the next. In other words, don't think about what you did well, might not have done so well or could have done even betterin a previous station. Part of what makes an applicant successful in this interview format is being able to move on quickly to the next station, refocus, and become immersed in the new station.

2. There is no right answer. If you don't have some information that might help you reach your conclusion, discuss that!

3. No knowledge is required for the MMI.

4. If an interviewer challenges your opinion, it is important to stay strong, show that you can consider his or her point of view and that you understand why he or she is challenging you. Whatever you do, don't let this throw you. Stay calm and unemotional and defend your opinion. Raters are instructed to challenge you.

5. The MMI is very difficult to prepare for. Even if you review and practice 500 scenarios, you will encounter new ones on your interview day! This means that you shouldn't memorize your responses and that you must keep an open

mind. Preparing well for the MMI is mostly about knowing what to expect so you aren't surprised by the structure and format of the interview.

6. While the MMI might sounds scary, surveys done in Canada and the UK have shown that applicants actually prefer this interview type over the traditional interview. In our anecdotal experience, our students often feel the same way or don't have a real preference.

7. You will never receive any feedback about how you did. You generally won't even get a smile or a nod. Interviewers are instructed to show zero emotion. This is sometimes very difficult for type-A medical school applicants.

8. Dress to impress. Be neat and tidy and dress like you'd want a doctor to dress!

9. Whenever possible, be kind, considerate, warm, approachable, compassionate, and empathetic.

PART 4:

SAMPLE MMI SCENARIOS

We advise you to use these sample scenarios for realistic practice by following these instructions.

Practice with a friend or family member who can give you feedback.

Read the prompt. Give yourself two minutes. Use a timer.

Offer your response. Give yourself eight minutes. Use a timer.

Tape your practice so you can listen and critique yourself.

If possible, dress in interview attire and have your friend/family member sit in an office and act as the rater.

Be sure your "rater" offers you no feedback or emotion during the encounter. He or she must remain straight faced.

Make sure you evaluate yourself not only on your response but also on your demeanor, body and facial language, posture, eye contact, and manners.

CHAPTER 29

MEDEDITS APPROACH TO ETHICAL
AND POLICY SCENARIOS

For ethical and policy related prompts, we suggest the following MedEdits approach we call SIMSLAC. By using this systematic approach, you will be sure to address everything that is needed in your response.

S - Summarize the prompt (and mentally figure out what type of prompt it is - ethical, cultural competence, professionalism, dealing with stress, teamwork, acting)

I - Issues - identify them

M - Missing or much-needed information - state what else could help you

S - Stakeholders - identify who and what are the most important players in the scenario

L - Life Experiences - talk about your own life experiences if you have any that relate to the discussion

A - Answer the question(s) being asked

C – Conclude your response

As you improve and practice offering your MMI responses, you will not need to follow this acronym methodically. However, when you first start preparing for your MMI, it will certainly help ensure that you don't leave out any necessary information in your discussion.

CHAPTER 30

ETHICAL AND POLICY SCENARIOS

SAMPLE SCENARIO #1:

During your first semester of medical school, your anatomy team (5 students to 1 cadaver) is holding a review session on Thursday evening for the big midterm on Friday. Your cousin's wedding is that weekend (out of town) and you had planned to attend – leaving Thursday and returning Sunday. What will you do?

Using the MedEdits SIMSLAC approach, let's work through this somewhat easy scenario step by step.

FIRST, YOU WILL SUMMARIZE THE PROMPT:

As I understand it, I am a member of an anatomy team and we have a huge exam on Friday. Yet I had already planned to go away for my cousin's wedding, which would result in my missing a review session on Thursday as well as the midterm on Friday. Is this correct?

Here the applicant does two things. First, she summarizes the prompt quite well to make sure she fully understands what is going on. Then, at the end of her summary, she "checks in" with her interviewer to make sure she is on track. Doing this type of check in satisfies two objectives. The interviewee makes sure she is on track and also sets the stage for possible dialogue with her rater, which can break the ice and make for a more comfortable and less stressful interview experience.

2) NEXT, IDENTIFY THE ISSUES.

It seems to me that several issues are at play here. First of all, I have an obligation to my team to contribute to the review session. As a team member, I would like to contribute to our work towards the midterm preparation. I also have an obligation to myself and the medical school. Making up an anatomy final would be a major headache (I would think). More important, as a medical student I am serious about my education and wouldn't want to miss such an important exam.

Here our applicant identifies the issues, acknowledges her responsibility to her team mates, and illustrates that she is serious about her studies and wants to do well.

3) IN THIS NEXT STEP, OUR STUDENT SEEKS OUT MORE INFORMATION THAT WILL HELP HER DECIDE HOW TO PROCEED.

I would like to know how far it is to my cousin's wedding from my medical school. Would it be possible to go to the review session and the exam and travel to the wedding on Friday night? I'd also like to know if I have committed to anything at the wedding. Am I a bridesmaid? Did I offer to help her with something on Thursday? If so, is there someone else who can help with those tasks?

Our student asks more questions and lets the rater know that she can think through this scenario and ask the questions that will help her make an informed decision about what to do. The rater may or may not offer answers to these questions but, by recognizing she doesn't have all of the information, the student shows she's able to see all sides of the situation.

4) WHO ARE THE STAKEHOLDERS?

If I left school on Thursday, I'd be letting my teammates down and I'd also be creating more work for my anatomy professor, who would need to help me make up the test. I would also be potentially compromising my own academic success and reputation. If I go to the wedding later than I had originally planned, I am potentially hurting my cousin, perhaps creating more work for someone else if I have committed to helping with the wedding.

Here our student clearly identifies everyone who might be affected by her decisions, including people not named in the scenario. She shows she can see the impact of her decision on many people and, in doing so, demonstrates her selflessness and empathy.

5) LIFE EXPERIENCES.

I actually had a similar experience recently. My good friend was having an engagement party that just happened to fall on the night I had to travel to New Orleans to present my research poster at a national meeting. This was a very important meeting that was the culmination of a year of work. I felt badly about hurting my friend; the party was really important to her. But then I told her I'd take her out for a nice lunch in the city on my own to celebrate.

By demonstrating she has been in a similar situation in her own life, our student demonstrates her commitment to her work and career. She also shows she's able to reach compromises and that friendships are important to her.

6) ANSWER

My responsibility to my classmates and my education must come first. I would do everything in my power to explain this situation empathetically to my cousin and that I would hope to travel to the wedding on Friday after the final. If I had any responsibilities related to the wedding, I would find out who could take them over to avoid stressing my cousin.

Our student gives a clear and unwavering response to the question that was asked of her (always pay attention to what is actually being asked of you). Her rater might challenge her on this response but she knows not to waver.

7) CONCLUSION

I think my decision would satisfy all involved parties and would not compromise my own success or that of my classmates or my cousin's wedding.

A quick concluding phrase to wrap it all up is a great way to end a response!

SAMPLE SCENARIO #2:

Your friend, who recently had spinal surgery, calls you to say that he is in a lot of pain and has run out of his Percocet (a narcotic pain medicine) and can't get in touch with his doctor. He asks you to please write him a prescription so he can get rid of his pain. How do you handle this situation? Would you prescribe the medication?

SUMMARY

My friend, who recently had surgery is in severe pain and is asking if I can write a prescription for pain medication because he can't reach his doctor. Is that correct?

Our student gives a nice quick summary of the easy- to- digest prompt.

2) ISSUES

This scenario presents several issues. First of all, my friend is in pain and I am concerned about that. However, I also think that the pain medicine he is taking could be addictive, and I have no idea when he finished his last prescription or how much medication he had. Finally, as a physician, I can't hand out prescriptions to anyone who asks; my license and professional reputation are at stake.

Our student goes through all of the issues related to this situation, showing understanding for her friend, acknowledging his pain and the possible consequences of taking too much of the medication. She also recognizes her own responsibility not to abuse her ability to prescribe medications and acknowledges that doing so could make things even worse for her friend.

3) MISSING OR MUCH NEEDED INFORMATION

To make a decision, I'd want to know when and how much medication my friend received from his doctor and when he finished it. I would also like to know if there is a doctor on call who can help my friend, access his medical history, and prescribe the medication. It is possible he is due for more.

By letting the rater know what other information she needs, the interviewee shows she recognizes that this problem might have other solutions that the prompt did not present,

4) STAKEHOLDERS

I need to consider several people: my friend who is in pain, his doctor who initially prescribed the medication, and me.

Here our applicant succinctly identifies all of the parties with a stake in this scenario. She recognizes that the doctor on call, who might also get involved in the situation but isn't even mentioned in the scenario, is not a stakeholder.

5) LIFE EXPERIENCES.

Because our student could not think of any life experiences that related to this scenario, she did not include this in her response.

6) ANSWER

As a physician, my first responsibility is to make sure my friend is okay. I would ask if I could visit him to make my own decision about his pain. Then I would recommend that he call his doctor's office to find out if there is anyone on call who could give him the medication. Since my friend is not actually my patient and because I don't know his history, I would not prescribe the medication, but I would help him find out who could help relieve his suffering. I thought about calling his doctor myself, but I don't want to violate his trust or confidentiality since the doctor may not know that my friend is seeking out pain medication from his friends.

This is a beautiful and well thought out answer that addresses all of the issues. Our respondent shows understanding, empathy, consideration of others, a willingness to help, the importance of patient/friend confidentiality, and that she won't betray her friend's trust. A good general rule to follow in any MMI scenario is never to leave a person in need and always to be an ally.

7) CONCLUSION

In summary, I would do whatever I could to make sure my friend wasn't suffering, helping him to get the care he needs but without violating my own professional and ethical code of conduct.

This is an excellent conclusion that neatly summarizes our interviewee's actions.

SAMPLE SCENARIO #3:

Your 36-year-old cousin, who is positive for the BRCA (breast cancer) gene, has just been diagnosed with stage 2 breast cancer, meaning the cancer is still contained within the breast. Your cousin tells you she does not believe in traditional medicine and is refusing the treatment her doctor advises. Instead, she plans to drink "anti-angiogenic" organic green juices hourly and walk barefoot in the grass to absorb the earth's vibrations and stimulate her immune system. What do you do? Would you try to convince her to choose traditional or alternative therapies?

SUMMARY

As I understand the prompt, my cousin has a recent diagnosis of breast cancer and would rather use alternative medicine than more traditional medical therapies. Is this correct?

Our applicant quickly summarizes the prompt and asks the rater to verify that she is on target.

ISSUES

There are several concerning issues here. First of all, I want the best for my cousin. As someone who believes in traditional therapy, and because it seems she is a high risk patient, I would encourage her to follow her doctor's orders. Assuming my cousin understands the risks of refusing therapy, however, neither I nor her doctor can force her to accept the recommended traditional therapies. At the same time, the "treatment" plan she has decided to follow is unlikely to be therapeutic.

Here the interviewee clearly states the issues, recognizing that her cousin has the right to refuse treatment and cannot be forced to engage in treatments to which she has not consented .

MISSING OR MUCH NEEDED INFORMATION

I would want to know if my cousin has been told about the benefits and risks of treatment. Has she read the literature and does she know about her chances of survival with traditional therapies? Does she know which of an array of traditional therapies are options for her type of disease? Has she looked into the alternative therapies in which she's interested ? Are there any data to support what she wants to do? I would also want to know if the alternative therapies might be harmful in any way.

By asking the right questions, our student targets the missing information that might allow her cousin to make an informed decision. Perhaps her cousin hasn't actually reviewed any data and has a doctor who doesn't supply the information that would answer these questions. In asking the right questions, the interviewee shows that her cousin may be making a decision without all of the information she needs.

STAKEHOLDERS

As a relative, I have the best interests of my cousin in the forefront of my mind. Her doctor does as well. I would also want my cousin to consider her loved ones and children, if she has any. For whom else is she responsible? Her decision about how to treat her breast cancer will impact many people besides herself.

Bringing up the obvious stakeholders, herself, the cousin, and her doctor, are great and our applicant goes beyond this to recognize that every decision a patient makes influences many others.

LIFE EXPERIENCES

The student has no life experiences that relate to this prompt and so skips this part of the analysis.

ANSWER

When talking to my cousin, I would explain my concern that she might be rejecting the therapy that would lead to the best outcome. I would encourage her to speak with her doctor to get the information and data she needs to make an informed decision. I would also offer to help her gather that data. We could do literature searches or even get a second opinion. After we collected all of the information I would then sit down with her and try to reason through everything in an intelligent and logical way. Assuming the traditional therapies showed better outcomes, I would advise her to choose the traditional route. Or, assuming the alternative therapy wasn't dangerous according to her doctor, I'd suggest she pursue the nontraditional therapies in conjunction with the traditional.

This response shows that our student is smart, a great critical thinker, and someone who is empathic and understanding. He doesn't judge his cousin for wanting to choose an alternative therapy, but instead seeks out the information he will need so his cousin can make an educated decision. He becomes his cousin's advocate and ally in this process.

CONCLUSION

In conclusion, I would suggest my cousin follow her doctor's orders, but I would also allow her to come to that decision on her own by collecting the available evidence to support that choice.

Short, sweet, and smart conclusion!

SAMPLE SCENARIO #4:

A patient you are seeing for the first time was just diagnosed with stomach cancer at an outside institution. The patient is not aware of her diagnosis. As you are about to walk in the room to evaluate and speak to your patient, the patient's son stops you and says, "Please don't tell my mother about her diagnosis. In our culture, we do not tell our family members when they have a dire medical problem so I ask you to please keep this information from her." How would you approach this situation? Would you tell the patient about her diagnosis?

SUMMARY

To summarize, a patient was recently diagnosed with cancer, but the patient's son doesn't want to tell his mom about the cancer because this deviates from their cultural norms.

Our student quickly summarizes the case.

ISSUES

The issues here are that the patient has a right to know about her diagnosis, prognosis, and treatment options and I, as her doctor, have an ethical and legal obligation to be completely honest with her. However, at the same time I don't want to contradict what is best for this patient from a cultural standpoint.

The student immediately recognizes that the patient has rights and that as her physician she is obligated to be honest. However, she also sees that this patient's cultural norms might affect how she advises this patient.

MISSING OR MUCH NEEDED INFORMATION

I would want to know, and I would ask the patient, how much she wanted to know. I would also like to better understand what the cultural norms were for this patient and her family. To do that, I might seek out the guidance of a social worker. An attorney might help me better understand my legal obligations. If the patient doesn't want to know about her diagnosis, am I required to tell her?

These are all great questions that show our student recognizes that she doesn't know everything and that she might need the help of outside professionals and experts. Knowing when to ask for help is the sign of a great doctor. Asking questions during an MMI is a wonderful way to demonstrate that you are thinking and can cope with not having the "right" answer immediately all of the time.

STAKEHOLDERS

I would have to consider what is in my patient's best interest, my best interest, and the interests of her son and extended family.

Our student clearly recognizes the stakeholders in the case. Once you become more adept at answering MMI questions, you might not need to state every stakeholder in this way, given that all three of these parties have been mentioned previously.

LIFE EXPERIENCES

It is not unusual for an applicant to have no life experiences related to this type of medical and policy case. This was the situation here.

ANSWER

In this situation and with the information I have, I would talk to the patient, get a full medical history, and explain to her that the son asked that I not discuss particular aspects of her case with her. I would ask her if that was okay with her. Depending on what she says, I would either disclose her diagnosis or not. Either way, I would make sure to see the patient again, very soon, once I was able to gather more information from the social worker and attorney.

Again, our student recognizes that she can make a clear cut decision only once she has more information. She also shows cultural sensitivity by basing her actions on the actual patient encounter. She also recognizes the importance of seeing this patient again.

CONCLUSION

To summarize, if the patient told me she didn't want to know specifics about her case, I would respect her wishes and wouldn't tell her. But, if she asked questions and wanted to know more or told me that she wanted to know everything, I wouldn't withhold any information from her.

The student offers two answers - one for each possible scenario outcome. Proposing different outcomes and asking questions during the MMI demonstrated our applicant's ability to think critically. Rarely can medical ethics cases be wrapped up in a bow. Many considerations must be taken into account, and you want to show that you are able to see multiple sides of any given issue. Our applicant did a great job here.

SAMPLE SCENARIO #5:

You are an emergency physician and have a patient who is having a myocardial infarction (heart attack). You ask the cardiologist on call to come in and evaluate the patient. When the cardiologist arrives, he is disheveled, has alcohol on his breath, and is slurring some words. Discuss how you would handle this situation. Would you report the cardiologist for arriving at the hospital drunk?

SUMMARY

I am a doctor in the emergency room and my patient is having a heart attack. The cardiologist who will also be taking care of my patient seems to be drunk.

This summary is straightforward.

ISSUES

The issues here are that my patient is really sick and needs care from a cardiologist. But, the cardiologist has been drinking so I am concerned about the care the he might be capable of giving my patient.

This is a short summary of the issues, which is fine. As you will see, our student elaborates further on these issues when he discusses his own life experiences. Scenarios dealing with alcohol or substance abuse are common in MMI interviews.

MISSING OR MUCH NEEDED INFORMATION

I would want to know if there was someone else on call who could take care of my patient.

Again, understanding when and how to use outside resources is important. The student realizes his patient needs a cardiologist, and the one who has arrived won't be able to care for the patient.

STAKEHOLDERS

I am faced with several considerations. First, I want the best care for my patient. I am also concerned about the cardiologist who seems drunk. As a medical professional, why would he be so irresponsible and put a patient's well being in jeopardy? I am also worried about my own and the hospital's liability. If I let this cardiologist care for my patient, knowing he is drunk, am I as guilty of bad judgment, and how would my mistake impact my hospital? Finally, I am putting the cardiologist's career in jeopardy, too. If he cares for this patient while he is drunk, he might make a crucial mistake. Also, if I report him that might put his career in jeopardy.

The interviewee does a great job going beyond the obvious in answering this question. She recognizes that she might be hurting not only the patient by allowing this cardiologist to care for her patient, but, she'd be hurting the cardiologist and the hospital. She recognizes that reporting her colleague might hurt his career.

LIFE EXPERIENCES

I recently went to a party where I met a friend who had been drinking. He said he was leaving and that he was driving home. I told him I felt that was dangerous, but he insisted he was okay. I tried to tell him that I would drive because I hadn't had anything to drink but he refused to let me. So, I grabbed his keys and would not give them back. He was really angry at me but thanked me later.

With life experiences to show that she has "done the right thing" in the past and understands that her answer might not be well received by the cardiologist, our applicant offers a great example of how she has dealt with a similar situation in the past.

ANSWER

So, I feel it would be my responsibility to do what is best for the patient, even though it wouldn't be easy, I would do as I did with my friend. I would pull the cardiologist aside and tell him my concerns and that I would have to find someone else to take care of my patient. I realize he might get angry with me. I would seek out more information about his drinking and would tell him that it was my obligation to tell my boss that he came to the hospital drunk. I would do my best to find out if this was a pattern and, if I thought it was, I would feel obligated to report him to someone in a position higher than mine. I would also make sure he had a safe way to get home and I would let him know I am happy to help in any way I can.

Our student recognizes the need to be honest with the cardiologist while taking excellent care of him by making sure he has a ride home and offering to help further, as well as making sure her patient receives the best care.

CONCLUSION

Ultimately, as a doctor, I would have to do what was best for my patient even if this means that my colleague was upset with me and might face disciplinary action.

This is a great conclusion because it shows the applicant can make unpopular decisions and is comfortable with confrontation.

Now try these next scenarios with a friend or family member:

SAMPLE SCENARIO #6:

You are a resident and have a patient with severe muscle spasm. Your attending asks you to order 1 milligram of valium intravenously. Accidentally, you order 10 milligrams of valium. The nurse comes to tell you that 10 minutes after he gave the patent the valium, he was asleep. Realizing your mistake, the nurse assures you the medicine will wear off, the patient will wake up, and it is nothing to worry about. Talk about how you manage this scenario.

SUMMARY

ISSUES

MISSING OR MUCH NEEDED INFORMATION

STAKEHOLDERS

LIFE EXPERIENCES

ANSWER

CONCLUSION

SAMPLE SCENARIO #7:

A mother brings in her 6- year- old daughter, who is having a severe asthma attack and comes to the hospital for "a few breathing treatments." You explain to the mother that the child is so sick that she needs to be admitted to the hospital for treatment. The mother refuses to let her child stay, however, saying that this has happened before, and she can treat her daughter at home with the medications she has from her home country in Mexico, from where they recently came. What would you do in this situation?

SUMMARY

ISSUES

MISSING OR MUCH NEEDED INFORMATION

STAKEHOLDERS

LIFE EXPERIENCES

ANSWER

CONCLUSION

SAMPLE SCENARIO #8:

A hospital in North Carolina recently ended a 40 year contract with a large anesthesiology group. The hospital says it took this action to increase profits and decrease patient costs. The anesthesiology group is concerned that this change will compromise patient care because the physician anesthesiologists probably will be replaced with nurse anesthetists. Talk about the issues involved.

SUMMARY

ISSUES

MISSING OR MUCH NEEDED INFORMATION

STAKEHOLDERS

LIFE EXPERIENCES

ANSWER

CONCLUSION

SAMPLE SCENARIO #9:

Premature babies, fewer than 24 weeks gestation, have low survival rates, and those that do survive often have poor outcomes. Yet most of these babies receive extensive medical care and have prolonged stays in the intensive care unit. What are the issues involved?

SUMMARY

ISSUES

MISSING OR MUCH NEEDED INFORMATION

STAKEHOLDERS

LIFE EXPERIENCES

ANSWER

CONCLUSION

SAMPLE SCENARIO #10:

A patient has multiple medical problems, is 90 years old, and lives in a nursing home where she is bed bound. Claiming she is miserable and has no quality of life, she says repeatedly that she wants to die and asks that she be given the means to do so. Discuss.

SUMMARY

ISSUES

MISSING OR MUCH NEEDED INFORMATION

STAKEHOLDERS

LIFE EXPERIENCES

ANSWER

CONCLUSION

SAMPLE SCENARIO #11:

A terminally ill patient develops cataracts and requests he have cataract surgery before he dies so he can see his family. Talk about this scenario and the issues it presents.

SUMMARY

ISSUES

MISSING OR MUCH NEEDED INFORMATION

STAKEHOLDERS

LIFE EXPERIENCES

ANSWER

CONCLUSION

CHAPTER 31
ACTING SCENARIOS

SAMPLE SCENARIO #12:

You are about to walk into a party with your friend. You have been looking forward to this party after a week of final exams. Your friend is in the room (meaning the actor, your "friend," is in the room).

Always try to start acting scenarios with an open ended statement and then a question, when possible. You won't always know what's coming, as is the case with this scenario, so go with the flow!

> **You:** I am so excited for this party. I think it'll be really fun. What do you think?

> **Friend:** Um. I'm not sure. Can we just stay in the car a little longer?

> **You:** Sure. Are you feeling okay? We can stay here for as long as you need. Is there anything you want to talk about?

In acting scenarios, always show sensitivity by asking for more information that might allow you to help more effectively.

> **Friend:** Honestly, I'm not great. I've never told you this before, but I really hate parties and groups. I get so nervous. My heart is racing.

> **You:** Oh gosh. I am so sorry you are feeling that way. How can I help you?

Our student immediately recognizes that her friend is anxious and needs time and security. She therefore doesn't push her friend to go into the party she's been looking forward to. Instead, she is patient with her friend and immediately offers to help. She makes the friend feel like she has an ally, which is comforting.

> **Friend:** I really don't know. I sometimes have bad social anxiety.

> **You:** I've learned about deep breathing exercises for anxiety because I went through a time when I was really anxious. Should we try that? I can guide you.

Our student first shows empathy for her friend and then offers a solution to help ease her friend's anxiety. This shows she understands how her friend feels.

> **Friend.** Okay. What do we do?

> **You:** Close your eyes. Now take in a deep breath while you are counting to 10. Then release the breath slowly. Focus

only on your breathing. Nothing else.

Friend: (tries the exercise).

You: Great. Now do it again.

Friend: (does the exercise again).

You: I find this helps when I get nervous. Do you want to keep doing it until you feel better? I will stay here.

Friend: I feel a little better, actually.

You: That's great. Do you want to try and go to the party? I will stay with you to make sure you feel okay. I find that sometimes when I confront my fears it helps me get over them.

Again, our student puts her friend before herself. She offers to stay with her friend, letting her know she can rely on her.

Friend: Sure. I can try. Are you sure you won't leave me?

You: No. I won't leave you. If you feel anxious again, tell me or give me a signal. I can also drive you home.

Friend: Thank you. Let's go.

Acting scenarios like this often end with a good resolution.

Now grab a friend or family member and work through these additional acting scenarios on your own.

SAMPLE SCENARIO #13:

You are the physician in charge of a busy medical practice. A patient comes in after falling off a ladder. The staff physician evaluates the patient and decides no diagnostic tests are needed and that the patient can be discharged. However, the patient is irate and insists he needs a CAT scan of his head. The staff physician refuses, saying the CAT scan is not warranted. Infuriated, the patient demands to speak with the physician in charge. What do you say to the patient?

SAMPLE SCENARIO #14:

You are a college student working on a group project. One member of your group, Alex, has not been contributing to the project and is not completing the tasks for which he is responsible. The rest of your teammates are getting really upset with Alex, saying that they are sick of doing all of his work. You volunteer to speak with Alex on behalf of the group. What do you say to him?

SAMPLE SCENARIO #15:

You are driving and, even though you know you shouldn't be doing this, you respond to a text you receive while stopped at a red light. You mistakenly take your foot off the brake and rear end the car in front of you. The driver, visibly irate, emerges from the car and is walking to your car while yelling that he is calling the police. What do you say to this man?

SAMPLE SCENARIO #16:

A department store at which you work has a liberal return policy. The store will accept any return item for an unlimited time as long as the customer has a return receipt. A customer brings in an item and she has a receipt. However, on closer inspection you notice that the tag on the item indicates it was purchased from another store. What do you say to this customer?

SAMPLE SCENARIO #17:

You are in anatomy lab getting ready to leave for the day when you overhear a friend bragging about posting a "cool picture" of his cadaver on Instagram. What do you say to your friend?

PART 5:

POST INTERVIEW AND FOLLOW UP

After a medical school interview, you want to take notes about everything you observed and everyone you met during your interview day. If you have multiple interviews, the specific experiences and observations you have may become muddled. Also write down the name and contact information for each of your one on one interviewers. You will need this later!

We first suggest that you follow any specific rules a medical school may have regarding post interview follow up and communications. Some medical school request that students don't write thank you notes, letters of intent, or letters of interest. In contrast, more and more schools actually request update letters and letters of intent. The majority of medical schools that do allow communication prefer you send them via email; however, some have online portals to submit additional information and others request only snail mail paper communications. Whatever a school's contact policy, be sure you adhere to it! You should be able to find this information on a medical school's website or the school may send you follow up information after your interview day.

CHAPTER 32
THANK YOU NOTES

For MMI interviews, we discourage trying to follow up and thank every "rater" you have during your interview. However, many MMI interviews, as I have mentioned before, are actually hybrid interviews with traditional stations. As a general rule, it is best to formally thank anyone with whom you have had a one on one interview or anyone with whom you truly connected during the interview day. Because handwritten thank you notes are one way lines of communication and typically end up in the garbage, we recommend email thank you notes. Why? There is always the possibility of having your interviewer reply to your email, which can establish dialogue. This can be especially helpful if you end up on a wait list at a top choice school. Assuming your interviewer replied to your thank you note, you can then "hit the reply" button once you are waitlisted to reiterate your interest in the medical school with the hope that your interviewer will advocate for you. Many of our students have had success using this approach. However, if your interviewer does not reply to an email thank you note, don't stress. We have had plenty of applicants write thank you emails without a reply who are subsequently accepted. We advise you to send email thank you notes within 48 hours of your interview.

Thank you notes to your interviewers will not influence your candidacy, but it is good manners to write them. Ideally, your notes should be concise yet should touch on some aspect of your interview that was unique. You should also mention something that you like about the school that relates to your interests and the topics discussed during your interview. Just like other aspects of this process, your note should reflect the tone of your interview. For example, if you had a great connection with an interviewer, your note might be longer and more personal. But, if your interview was brief and superficial, you might only mention specific things you like about the school.

EXAMPLE-- THANK YOU NOTE #1:

Dear Dr. XXX,

Thank you very much for taking the time to interview me on November 5th. I really enjoyed meeting you and learning about Academic Medical School. I think that Academic would be a great fit for me. I appreciate the new integrated curriculum and feel that this suits my learning style. I am also intrigued by the opportunity to work at the student run clinic, which would allow me to continue helping the underserved. I hope your lecture at the National Society of Esteemed Faculty went well.

I would be honored to learn from you as a student at Academic. If there is anything else you need to evaluate my candidacy, please let me know.

Best regards,
Prospective Student
AAMC ID: (always offer this for easy look up!)

WHAT DOES THIS STUDENT DO?

- Thanks the interviewer for his time
- Mentions the new curriculum
- Mentions his interest in the underserved
- Brings up something that was discussed at the interview
- Offers to provide additional information

EXAMPLE-- THANK YOU NOTE #2:

Dear Dr. Paris,

I wanted to thank you for spending time with me on my interview day. I really enjoyed learning about Top Medical School and feel it would be a great fit for me. Because of my interest in working with refugee populations, I value the patient populations that Top Hospitals serve and the chance to rotate not only in the city, but in the surrounding suburbs and smaller cities as well. It was great to learn about our mutual interests in public health, and I think you'd be an ideal mentor for me if I were lucky enough to attend Top. I also really liked all of the medical students I met and feel I would fit in well with the student body. Please feel free to get in touch if you have any questions.

Thank you again.

Sincerely,
Sarah Smile
AAMC ID: (always offer this for easy look up!)

WHAT DOES THIS STUDENT DO?

- Thanks the interviewer for his time
- Mentions her interest in refugee populations
- Mentions the hospitals where she will rotate
- Brings up something that was discussed at the interview
- Offers to provide additional information

The key to a thank you note is to identify what you value about the medical school where you interviewed (you can mention location, too) and to touch on something you discussed with the interviewer if that is possible. Do not "try too hard" when you write thank you notes. Simple and straightforward is better than over the top and contrived. As in the interview itself, authenticity is paramount. By the same token, don't be too casual in your writing and stay away from slang and abbreviations. Your thank you notes should be formal, brief letters to express your gratitude and interests. No thank you note will ever change an admissions decision; these notes are really just a way to communicate that you are a respectful, gracious, and kind person.

CHAPTER 33

THE WAITLIST (PARTS EXCERPTED FROM THE MEDEDITS GUIDE TO MEDICAL SCHOOL ADMISSIONS, THIRD EDITION)

If you are waitlisted at a top choice school, you can influence your chance of being accepted off a wait list by writing a letter of intent (see the next chapter). You can also send in additional letters of recommendation (ideally from new medical writers) assuming the medical school(s) at which you are waitlisted allow this. For students who are still in college or taking classes, these additional letters of reference can come from professors. Many students also send in letters from a new principal investigator, research supervisor, or work supervisor.

Most schools will not reveal exactly how many applicants they "waitlist" (some are, literally, 400 people deep), but most will tell you what percentage of their class "comes off the waitlist." In general, more competitive schools take fewer people off the waitlist since at top schools up to 75% of applicants who are accepted actually attend, compared with 35% at less competitive schools.

Most waitlists are non-rolling, and schools will consider waitlist applicants only after April 30th when all accepted students can hold only one acceptance. (See "If I am accepted to another school, what happens if I get off a waitlist at a school I would rather attend?")

For medical schools that start classes before July 30th, however, you must hold only this acceptance as of April 15th. Some medical schools have "rolling waitlists" that are considered throughout the interview season. Some waitlists are ranked while others are not. Most schools will let you know their waitlist procedures if you are placed on their waitlist. (See "Important dates for medical school applicants")

IF I AM ACCEPTED TO ANOTHER SCHOOL, WHAT HAPPENS IF I GET OFF A WAITLIST AT A SCHOOL I WOULD RATHER ATTEND?

You are allowed to accept a waitlist acceptance until you have matriculated in medical school. So, let's say you are accepted to medical school A but really want to attend medical school B where you are waitlisted. If medical school B offers you a spot off the waitlist, you can withdraw from medical school A and attend medical school B as long as you have not yet matriculated at medical school A. What does matriculate mean? This means that you have already started classes, which usually means having begun orientation.

IMPORTANT DATES FOR MEDICAL SCHOOL APPLICANTS

October 15 : Medical schools can extend acceptances after this date.

March 15: MD/PhD programs must extend a number of acceptances that is at least equal to the number of students in the matriculating class.

March 15: Medical schools must extend a number of acceptances that is at least equal to the number of students in the matriculating class.

April 30: MD and MD/PhD applicants can hold only one acceptance. Applicants can accept waitlist offers before they matriculate.

April 30th: Medical school applicants may hold only one acceptance to medical school. They can accept waitlist offers before they matriculate at the medical school where they are holding a spot. Before April 30th, students may hold multiple acceptances by submitting refundable deposits to medical schools

After April 30th, schools may require students to respond to acceptance offers in five business days or less.

No medical school or program is allowed to extend an acceptance offer to a student once he or she has already started orientation or is enrolled in classes at another medical school.

CHAPTER 34
LETTER OF INTENT AND LETTER OF INTEREST (PARTS EXCERPTED FROM THE MEDEDITS GUIDE TO MEDICAL SCHOOL ADMISSIONS, THIRD EDITION)

If you are waitlisted at your top choice school, the best thing you can do is to send a letter of intent that clearly states that you will attend the medical school if accepted. For medical schools where you have not yet received an interview but hope to, consider sending a letter of interest. The only difference between a letter of intent and a letter of interest is that a letter of intent clearly states that the school is your number one choice whereas a letter of interest does not. Letters of intent and interest should also include any updates you might have regarding your recent accomplishments and experiences. More and more medical schools are actually asking waitlisted applicants to express interest in writing. So, letters of intent are becoming more important than they were in the past.

Sending a letter of intent to the top choice school where you are waitlisted is extremely important. Clearly express that the medical school is your #1 choice and that you will attend if accepted. You should also be specific about why you are interested in the medical school and try to relate those interests to your background and accomplishments. You should also update medical schools on any recent accomplishments. It also is wise to send additional letters of reference from professors or supervisors if this is an option. More support of your candidacy is always helpful.

Why are letters of intent important? Medical schools have several reasons for wanting to accept people whom they know will attend. First, medical schools want enthusiastic students who will add to the morale of the student body. They also like to know, especially as the date of matriculation nears, that the applicant they accept will attend; no medical school wants an open seat on the first day of classes. Finally, medical schools like the percentage of accepted applicants who matriculate to be as high as possible since this reflects the competitiveness of the medical school.

SAMPLE LETTERS OF INTENT

EXAMPLE-- LETTER OF INTENT #1

Dear Dr. XXX (Address this to the dean of admissions or the director of admissions, depending on the school's instructions):

I am a current applicant at The Awesome Medical School and interviewed there on October 25th. I am writing this letter to reiterate that AMC is my top choice for medical school and to update you on my accomplishments since my interview. If accepted, I would withdraw my other medical school applications and attend Awesome Medical School.

AMC will help me achieve my goal to one day become an excellent academic emergency physician. I hope to continue my research with Dr. Smart on the use of the novel new biomarker, C2D, for diagnosing a myocardial infarction. Dr. Smart currently is conducting this research in the emergency department. Additionally, since I have an avid interest in early goal-directed therapy because my grandmother died of sepsis and multiorgan failure two years ago, I look forward to working with intensive care physicians to learn more about this topic. With the many hospitals and free clinics that surround AMC, I will also be able to continue my work with helping the underserved. As a medical student, I will strive to be knowledgeable and compassionate and to make a meaningful contribution to the school.

Since my interview, I earned straight As in all my courses. I have also received a prestigious research award at my college. I have helped write a manuscript summarizing my research in the emergency department, which will be submitted for publication. I was named a Sherwood Scholar at my college because of the challenging workload I undertook and the grades I earned. I was also recognized by my peers through a Peer Achievement Award, which is awarded annually to two graduating seniors.

Thank you very much for considering my candidacy. I would be honored to attend AMC and hope to be accepted.

Sincerely,

A Future Medical Student
AAMC ID: (always include this for easy lookup!)

EXAMPLE-- LETTER OF INTENT #2

Dear Dr. Take Me,

I am writing this letter to update you on my accomplishments since I interviewed at Great School of Medicine in September. Since my interview, I have had interviews at several other medical schools and now know that Great is the perfect fit for me. If accepted to Great, I will attend.

As I discussed with Dr. Wish on my interview day, I have a commitment to help the underserved. I was impressed by the student run clinic at Great and was also intrigued by the number of faculty who are committed to helping the underserved. I feel that Great would provide me with role models who will help me develop into the type of doctor I hope to become.

I could also pursue my interest in neuroscience at Great. My undergraduate neuroscience research has been one of my most significant achievements as an undergraduate. Dr. Neuro, at Great, studies the same type of neurosynapses on which I have focused as an undergraduate. The neurology research together with the outstanding neurology department at Great would allow me to explore my interest in the specialty and establish my niche while still a medical student.

Finally, I really enjoyed meeting the current medical students on my interview day. They are bright, interesting, and supportive of each other. I can see myself fitting in very well at Great.

If accepted to Great, I will take advantage of the resources and opportunities available to me to hone the skills I need to become a great physician. I will work hard to become a valuable member of my medical school class and make a meaningful contribution.

Thank you for your consideration. If I am offered a position in the Great Medical School incoming class, I will enthusiastically accept it.
Best regards,

Aspiring Doctor
AAMC ID: (always include this for easy lookup!)

EXAMPLE-- LETTER OF INTEREST #1

Dear Dean of Admissions,

I am an applicant to Stan Medical School and remain hopeful that I will receive an interview. I am writing this letter to express my sincere interest in Stan and update you about my recent accomplishments. Dr. Tan, my research advisor, has also offered to write me an additional letter of reference, which you should be receiving soon.

This year I have been working with Dr. Tan on a clinical research study at Better Than You Medical School on clinical trials studying the impact of a new drug for amyloid patients suffering from cardiac manifestations of the disease. I am not allowed to discuss our findings thus far, but what we have discovered offers great promise for this population of patients. I really enjoy not only working with Dr. Tan and the rest of our research team but also working with the patients and their families and helping them cope with this disabling disease. I have gained so much insight about the patient experience and have also volunteered to be a part of our weekly patient support groups. This multidisciplinary experience has offered me insight about how hospitals operate, teamwork, and other specialities in medicine.

I also took an upper level immunology class at the University of Better (U of B) which built on what I studied as an undergraduate. I am happy to report that I earned an A in this class. I am currently taking a bioengineering class at U of B and thus far have an A in that class as well.

I would appreciate the opportunity to interview at Stan despite the fact that I am fortunate to already have a medical school acceptance. Stan's amyloid team would allow me to continue exploring my interest in this disease. I also value Stan's case-based approach to learning and the emphasis on simulation medicine throughout medical school. I would also love to live in Stan City which is close to my family.

I look forward to hearing from you.
Best,

Bill Morgan
AAMC ID: (always include this for easy lookup!)

APPENDIX A
MEDICAL SCHOOL INTERVIEW TYPE

Medical School Interview Type Listed by State (most updated list at the time this book was written. Subject to change.)

ALABAMA

University of Alabama School of Medicine
Traditional open file and Multiple mini interviews

University of South Alabama College of Medicine
Traditional open file

ARIZONA

University of Arizona College of Medicine
Multiple MiniInterviews

University of Arizona Phoenix
Multiple Mini Interviews

ARKANSAS

University of Arkansas for Medical Sciences College of Medicine
Blind team interviews

CALIFORNIA

California Northstate University School of Medicine
Multiple mini & group Interview

California University of Science and Medicine
Multiple mini interviews

Keck School of Medicine of the University of Southern California
Traditional closed file

Loma Linda University School of Medicine
Traditional open file

Stanford University School of Medicine
Multiple Mini Interview

University of California, Davis, School of Medicine
Multiple Mini Interviews

University of California, Irvine, School of Medicine
Traditional open file

University of California, Los Angeles David Geffen School of Medicine
Multiple Mini Interviews

University of California, Riverside, School of Medicine
Multiple Mini Interviews

University of California, San Diego School of Medicine

Multiple Mini Interviews

University of California, San Francisco, School of Medicine
Two closed file interviews

COLORADO
University of Colorado School of Medicine
Traditional open file

CONNECTICUT
Frank H. Netter MD School of Medicine at Quinnipiac University
Traditional open file

University of Connecticut School of Medicine
Traditional open file and group interview sessions

Yale School of Medicine
Traditional open file

DISTRICT OF COLUMBIA
Georgetown University School of Medicine
Traditional open file

George Washington University School of Medicine and Health Sciences
Traditional blind file

Howard University College of Medicine
Traditional open file

FLORIDA

Florida Atlantic University Charles E. Schmidt College of Medicine
Traditional open file & behavioral

Florida International University Herbert Wertheim College of Medicine
Traditional semi blind file

Florida State University College of Medicine
Traditional open file

University of Central Florida College of Medicine
Traditional partially blind file

University of Florida College of Medicine
Traditional partially blind file

University of Miami Leonard M. Miller School of Medicine
Traditional open file

USF Health Morsani College of Medicine
Traditional closed file interviews.

GEORGIA

Emory University School of Medicine
Traditional open file and group interview.

Medical College of Georgia at Georgia Regents University
Two traditional interviews. One closed and one open file.

Mercer University School of Medicine
Traditional open file interviews.

Morehouse School of Medicine
Traditional open file interviews

HAWAII
University of Hawaii, John A. Burns School of Medicine
Traditional open file interviews

ILLINOIS

Chicago Medical School at Rosalind Franklin University of Medicine & Science
Multiple Mini Interviews

Loyola University Chicago Stritch School of Medicine
Traditional semi-open file and closed file.

Northwestern University The Feinberg School of Medicine
Traditional open file interview and a panel interview

Rush Medical College of Rush University Medical Center
Traditional open file

Southern Illinois University School of Medicine
Traditional open file

University of Chicago Division of the Biological Sciences The Pritzker School of Medicine
Traditional open file interviews

University of Illinois College of Medicine
Traditional open file or panel.

INDIANA
Indiana University School of Medicine
Traditional open file

IOWA
University of Iowa Roy J. and Lucille A. Carver College of Medicine
Traditional open file and a case-based learning session

KANSAS
University of Kansas School of Medicine
Traditional open file

KENTUCKY
University of Kentucky
Traditional open file

University of Louisville School of Medicine
Traditionally partially blind interviews

LOUISIANA
Louisiana State University School of Medicine in New Orleans
Traditional open file

Louisiana State University School of Medicine in Shreveport
Traditional open and closed file

Tulane University School of Medicine

Traditional open file

MARYLAND

Johns Hopkins University School of Medicine
Traditional open file

Uniformed Services University of the Health Sciences F. Edward
Hebert School of Medicine
Traditional open file

University of Maryland School of Medicine
Traditional open file

MASSACHUSETTS

Boston University School of Medicine
Traditional open file

Harvard Medical School
Traditional open file

Tufts University School of Medicine
Traditional open file

University of Massachusetts Medical School
Multiple Mini Interviews

MICHIGAN

Central Michigan University College of Medicine
Multiple Mini Interviews

Michigan State University College of Human Medicine

Multiple Mini Interviews session and traditional open file with a student

Oakland University William Beaumont School of Medicine
Traditional open file

University of Michigan Medical School
Traditional open file
Several shorter interviews

Wayne State University School of Medicine
Traditional open file

Western Michigan University Homer Stryker M.D. School of Medicine
Traditional open file

MINNESOTA
Mayo Medical School
Traditional partially blind file

University of Minnesota Medical School
Traditional open file

MISSISSIPPI
University of Mississippi School of Medicine
Multiple Mini Interviews

MISSOURI
Saint Louis University School of Medicine
Traditional open file

University of Missouri-Columbia School of Medicine
Traditional open file

University of Missouri-Kansas City School of Medicine
Multiple Mini Interviews

Washington University in St. Louis School of Medicine
Traditional open file

NEBRASKA
Creighton University School of Medicine
Traditional open file.

University of Nebraska College of Medicine
Traditional open file

NEVADA
University of Nevada School of Medicine
Multiple Mini Interviews

NEW HAMPSHIRE
Geisel School of Medicine at Dartmouth
Traditional open file

NEW JERSEY
Cooper Medical School of Rowan University
Traditional open file and blind

Rutgers New Jersey Medical School
Traditional open file

Rutgers, Robert Wood Johnson Medical School
Multiple Mini Interviews

Seton Hall - Hackensack Meridian School of Medicine
Traditional open file

NEW MEXICO
University of New Mexico School of Medicine
Traditional open file

NEW YORK
Albany Medical College
Multiple Mini Interviews

Albert Einstein College of Medicine
Traditional open file

City University of New York School of Medicine
Traditional open file

Columbia University College of Physicians and Surgeons
Traditional open file

Hofstra North Shore - LIJ School of Medicine
Traditional open file

Icahn School of Medicine at Mount Sinai
Traditional open file

Jacobs School of Medicine and Biomedical Sciences at the
University at Buffalo

Traditional open file

New York Medical College
Multiple Mini Interviews

New York University School of Medicine
Multiple Mini Interviews

State University of New York Downstate Medical Center
College of Medicine
Traditional open file

Stony Brook University School of Medicine
Traditional open file

University of Rochester School of Medicine and Dentistry
Traditional open file and small group session

Duke University School of Medicine
Multiple Mini Interviews

State University of New York Upstate Medical University
Multiple Mini Interviews

Weill Cornell Medicine
Traditional open file

NORTH CAROLINA
Duke University School of Medicine
Multiple Mini Interviews

The Brody School of Medicine at East Carolina University
Traditional partially blind interviews

University of North Carolina at Chapel Hill School of Medicine
Traditional open file

Wake Forest School of Medicine of Wake Forest Baptist Medical
Center
Traditional open file

NORTH DAKOTA
University of North Dakota School of Medicine and Health
Sciences
Panel interview

OHIO
Case Western Reserve University School of Medicine
Traditional open file

Northeast Ohio Medical University
Traditional open file

Ohio State University College of Medicine
Traditional partially blind file

University of Cincinnati College of Medicine
Multiple Mini Interviews

The University of Toledo College of Medicine
Traditional open file

Wright State University Boonshoft School of Medicine
Traditional open file

OKLAHOMA
University of Oklahoma College of Medicine
Panel interview

OREGON
Oregon Health & Science University School of Medicine
Multiple Mini Interviews

PENNSYLVANIA
Drexel University College of Medicine
Traditional open file and group interview with students-closed-file

Lewis Katz School of Medicine at Temple University
Traditional open file

Pennsylvania State University College of Medicine
Traditional open file

Raymond and Ruth Perelman School of Medicine at the University of Pennsylvania
Traditional open file

Sidney Kimmel Medical College at Thomas Jefferson University
Traditional open file

The Commonwealth Medical College
Traditional open file

University of Pittsburgh School of Medicine
Traditional open file

PUERTO RICO
Ponce Health Sciences University School of Medicine
Traditional open file or group

San Juan Bautista School of Medicine
Traditional open file and Multiple Mini Interviews

Universidad Central del Caribe School of Medicine
Multiple Mini Interviews

University of Puerto Rico School of Medicine
Not available

RHODE ISLAND
The Warren Alpert Medical School of Brown University
Traditional open file and group

SOUTH CAROLINA
Medical University of South Carolina College of Medicine
Traditional open file

University of South Carolina School of Medicine
Traditional open file

University of South Carolina School of Medicine - Greenville
Traditional open file and one blind, and a 30 minute Multiple
Mini Interview session with 4 mini-interview stations.

SOUTH DAKOTA

Sanford School of Medicine The University of South Dakota
Traditional open file

TENNESSEE

East Tennessee State University James H. Quillen College of Medicine
Traditional open file

Meharry Medical College
Traditional open file

University of Tennessee Health Science Center College of Medicine
Traditional open file

Vanderbilt University School of Medicine
Traditional open file and closed file

TEXAS

Baylor College of Medicine
Traditional open file

Texas A&M Health Science Center College of Medicine
Traditional open file

Texas Tech University Health Sciences Center Paul L. Foster School of Medicine
Traditional open file

Texas Tech University Health Sciences Center School of

Medicine
Traditional open file

University of Texas at Austin Dell Medical School
Two Traditional Interviews, five MMI stations, one group problem solving exercise

University of Texas Medical Branch School of Medicine
Traditional open file

University of Texas Medical School at Houston
Traditional open file

University of Texas Rio Grande Valley School of Medicine
Two traditional interviews - one open and one blind

University of Texas Southwestern Medical Center at Dallas Southwestern Medical School
Traditional open file

UTAH
University of Utah School of Medicine
Multiple Mini Interview and traditional open file

VERMONT
University of Vermont College of Medicine
Multiple Mini Interviews

VIRGINIA
Eastern Virginia Medical School
Panel interviews.

University of Virginia School of Medicine
Traditional open file

Virginia Commonwealth University School of Medicine
Multiple Mini Interviews

Virginia Tech Carilion School of Medicine
Multiple Mini-Interview consists of one traditional interview and a series of nine scenario stations.

WEST VIRGINIA
Marshall University Joan C. Edwards School of Medicine
Traditional open file

West Virginia University School of Medicine
Traditional open file

WISCONSIN
Medical College of Wisconsin
Traditional open file

University of Wisconsin School of Medicine and Public Health
Traditional open file and a 45-minute small group discussion with other interviewees and current medical students.

APPENDIX B

QUESTIONS TO ASK THE
CURRENT MEDICAL STUDENTS

GENERAL

Are you happy?

Why did you choose to come here?

What are the best things about the school?

Do you think that what was presented to you on interview day was accurate?

How do you like living here?

CURRICULUM

What are the strengths and weakness of the curriculum? Do you know of any changes in the curriculum?

Are faculty supportive of student feedback regarding the curriculum?

CLINICAL ROTATIONS

What do you think of the clnical sites? Is there bedside teaching?

Is most teaching done by housestaff or faculty? What are the best/worst rotations here?

Are you learning how to practice evidence based medicine?

Do you think you have enough flexibility to choose elective rotations?

RESEARCH

Do most students do research?

Do you have to seek out opportunities on your own?

Teaching and mentoring

Do faculty and residents teach?

Do you have enough 1:1 time with residents and faculty?

Do faculty help with specialty selection and the match process?

STUDENT LIFE

How would you describe the camaraderie among students?

What do students do in their free time?

Where do students live?

How do most students get to school?

Do students participate in volunteer, community service, or teaching activities?

WANT MORE INFORMATION?

For more information about MedEdits' services including mock interviews, feel free to contact us: info@mededits.com or 646-217-4674.

Visit our website: www.MedEdits.com.

We would also value feedback on this book so we can modify future editions

Read other books by Dr. Freedman, including The MedEdits Guide to Medical School Admission, Third Edition

The MedEdits Guide to Medical Schools Admissions covers many topics including:

• Where to go to college if you are premed

- When to take the MCAT
- Retaking the MCAT
- Whom to ask for letters of reference and how
- How to improve your candidacy
- What medical schools look for in applicants
- How to decide what topics should be included in the application written materials
- How to approach the personal statement
- How to approach the application and most meaningful entries
- Applying to allopathic, osteopathic, off-shore, and Texas medical schools
- The different application systems: AMCAS, TMDSAS, and AACOMAS
- Deciding where to apply and attend
- Average GPAs and MCATs for accepted students
- What to do if you are waitlisted

The book includes multiple full length examples of:
Personal statements
- Application entries and "most meaningful" descriptions
- Secondary essays
- Letters of intent

Whether you are an outstanding candidate for acceptance to a top-tier allopathic medical school or are aspiring to get in anywhere, the no-nonsense advice this comprehensive guide offers will greatly improve your chances of achieving your goals

WHAT IS MEDEDITS, LLC?

OUR STORY

When Dr. Jessica Freedman, the founder of MedEdits Medical Admissions, was on faculty at the Icahn School of Medicine at Mount Sinai, she found great joy in advising and mentoring students and residents. This led her to leave Mount Sinai to launch MedEdits Medical Admissions in 2007. The demand for MedEdits services has grown during the past several years, leading to an expansion of our team, which now includes several experienced medical educators and physicians, all of whom have admissions experience, and a talented group of professional editors.

MedEdits Medical Admissions is recognized for superior one-on-one advising and editing services, a track record of success, and a unique collaborative advising approach. Our team's combined wisdom helps each student achieve the best results. Most of our clients now come to us by word of mouth, further evidence of our excellent reputation.

Our message is far reaching. Dr. Freedman has written four best-selling books on the medical admissions process and has been quoted in many media outlets. We have more than 50,000 followers on Facebook and Twitter. Yet we are committed to each and every student with whom we work, and our services are personalized and individually tailored. For more information, we encourage you to contact us.

PROVEN RESULTS

MedEdits has successfully helped hundreds of applicants through the medical school and residency admissions processes. Some are outstanding candidates while others are "borderline." We give every student individualized guidance based on his or her situation and background.

This year, more than 50,000 students applied to allopathic (MD) medical schools in the United States. Fewer than half of these students will be accepted to medical school.

By working with MedEdits, you can join our successful group of students; a remarkable 94% of MedEdits students who work with us on every part of the admissions process are accepted to allopathic medical schools in the United States. The vast majority (95%) of residency applicants who work with us comprehensively match in the specialty of their choice. Many match at their #1 choice. This doesn't mean we can work miracles, but it does mean that we can help students to devise a strategy that will make them the most competitive applicants possible. MedEdits' expertise and a well developed plan can yield phenomenal results.

EXPERTISE AND WISDOM

Dr. Freedman served on faculty at the Icahn School of Medicine at Mount Sinai where she worked in both residency leadership and served on the medical school admissions committee. She also worked at Elmhurst Hospital in Queens, New York, a major affiliate of Mount Sinai, with international medical graduates and Caribbean medical students. She has conducted hundreds of interviews and reviewed thousands of applications.

MedEdits consultants are all experienced academic faculty medical educators with admissions experience who pride themselves in providing support to, and working with, students. All of our consultants have served on medical admissions committees for at least five years and have made pivotal decisions about applicants' fates. Dr. Jessica Freedman has hand selected each consultant to ensure that he or she upholds MedEdits ideals by offering the most up to date guidance, based on knowledge and experience, with professionalism and warmth. All of our consultants are experienced medical educators. With MedEdits, you will not work with recent medical school graduates, current resident trainees, or individuals without extensive experience in academic medicine.

TOP MEDICAL SCHOOL ADMISSION CONSULTANTS

Our team is exceptional. It may be a cliché, but with regard to medical admissions counseling you do get what you pay for; be wary of working with an individual or company with less experience or lower fees than MedEdits; doing so may result in inferior service. A current medical student, a resident physician, a physician without faculty level medical school and residency admissions experience, or a company that offers professional editors but no one with medical admissions experience cannot offer the insight and wisdom that we can. No one in the industry has our breadth and depth of experience and insight. By working with MedEdits, you can be confident that you are giving your application to medical school, residency, or fellowship your absolute best shot. Hiring the best company is an investment in your future – so do your homework and choose wisely!

Every year we work with students who either weren't accepted to medical school or could have had better results or didn't get a residency because they chose to work with other individuals or companies who had less experience or because they chose to navigate this complicated process on their own. Don't make this mistake.

HOLISTIC MEDICAL SCHOOL, RESIDENCY, AND FELLOWSHIP ADVISING

MedEdits offers one-on-one individualized guidance and coaching. When clients start working with MedEdits, they complete a detailed questionnaire, which allows us to obtain a thorough applicant history. This offers us a comprehensive picture of the client's ideals and insights so we can then guide the client to create more compelling and thoughtful documents — a key to success.

Flexibility: Every student has his or her own story. We'll work with you.

We offer many different med school admissions consulting services depending on each client's needs. Applicants can choose to work with us on a short or long term basis and we provide services at multiple price points.

SUPERIOR DOCUMENT PREPARATION: PERSONAL STATEMENT, APPLICATION, AND ADMISSIONS DOCUMENTS

A professional MedEdits senior editor reviews every document submitted to MedEdits. MedEdits' unique essay coaching and editing process allows you to bring out the best of your candidacy in your own words and style. With our proven essay coaching techniques, we will ask thought provoking questions that will help you to think of ideas and insights that you probably wouldn't have thought of on your own. This allows you to create documents that will distinguish you, making the admissions officer interested and curious to learn more about your candidacy. We never write documents on behalf of clients, but we will inspire you to write to the best of your ability and in the most compelling fashion possible.

BEST MEDICAL SCHOOL CONSULTANTS: A COLLABORATIVE TEAM APPROACH

Because each MedEdits consultant and professional medical editor has a unique set of experiences, clients benefit from our pool of expertise. The medical admissions process has many nuances, and our team of experts are from different geographic areas and have worked at many outstanding medical schools throughout the country. We collaborate frequently, and this team philosophy offers a greater benefit to the applicant than if we each worked alone and in a vacuum. Our team, as a whole, takes great pride in the work we do, and this applicant-centered view defines our commitment to the clients we serve. MedEdits has the best medical school admissions advisors.

DEDICATION TO EVERY CLIENT

At MedEdits Medical Admissions, the nation's best medical school admissions advisors, we are fully devoted to our clients and are not distracted by outside commitments. Dr. Jessica Freedman, our company's founder, coordinates the work of all members of our team.

EVIDENCE-BASED ACADEMIC GUIDANCE

We attend the annual Association of American Medical Colleges meeting and read the academic medicine literature to stay up to date with the most recent statistics and data. This allows us to serve as a cutting edge resource. We also have regularly scheduled MedEdits faculty meetings to discuss students and trends in medical education.

CODE OF ETHICS

We hold ourselves to high ethical standards and maintain confidentiality.

MEDEDITS MEDICAL ADMISSIONS

WHAT OUR CLIENTS ARE SAYING:

"I want to thank you for helping me truly express my experiences and intentions on my application to medical school. I feel that without the opportunity to work with you I may not have had any success. I am so grateful for all of your input and encouragement and perhaps we will work together again when I am applying for residency! The elusive dream that I have always wanted to pursue but had to build up the confidence for over the past few years has finally come true. Thank you again for all your help....

-Medical School Applicant, California

"I got into Cornell for medical school. YEAH!!! Thanks for all your help. The money I paid you was definitely worth it. It has made everything so much easier, thus avoiding any horrible acne outbreaks. Yay!...
-Medical School Applicant, New York

"It seems that [our daughter] has decided on Harvard for medical school. Your help to her has been truly invaluable and my husband and I both felt a tremendous sense of comfort in knowing that you were there to give [our daughter] such "spot on" advice and we could just hang back and be parents through this very difficult and very very lengthy (seemingly endless) process…Once again, thank you again-you have been fantastic! Feel free to use us as references for other parents and I'm sure [our daughter] would be thrilled to be a reference as a student who has gone through the process. I'm sure she will be in touch before residency time!!!!! …

-Parent of Medical School Applicant, Florida

"I appreciate the kindness you have shown to [our child]; I know it is a business, but I really do appreciate the nature of the advice and assistance you have given to her. You really have made [our child] feel like she has an ally in this ordeal – and for that, I am personally grateful to you…

-Parent of Medical School Applicant, New Jersey

"I believe it was all because of your step by step guidance and coaching/mentoring that you provided [my son] over the course of the year, on how to put his best foot forward in various situations that he has had success. He now has acceptances from a number of medical schools and will soon make his choice. I am very appreciative of your help for him during the process and thank you for all you did for him...Thanks in advance, and I hope [my son] will turn back to you when he is starting to think about residency programs etc. Once again, thank you so very much and let me know if there is anything I can do for you...."

-Parent of Medical School Applicant, Michigan

"I got accepted to medical school! I definitely thought the interview preparation helped. At all schools I have been at I was noticeably less nervous than other applicants. I felt very confident and well-prepared thanks to your advice and encouragement! Thanks so much for all of your help. As a reapplicant, I really think you took my application to the next level with your advice and expert editing team! Dr. Freedman and her editing team helped turn a decent application into an excellent one, greatly enhancing my AMCAS® entries, personal statement, and even providing help on secondaries...."

-Medical School Applicant, Texas

"We appreciate all the help you have given our son, a medical school reapplicant, during the application process. We definitely feel your guidance helped him immensely. Both my son and I feel that your intimate knowledge of the medical school admissions process gave us a thorough and sound advice throughout the entirety of the application cycle, from filling out the AMCAS® to interview day. We definitely feel your help strengthened the AMCAS® application and your interview feedback provided the confidence to perform well no matter the school. Working with you definitely improved my son's chances of acceptance. [Follow up: son will matriculate at a top US medical school.]…

-Parent of Medical School Applicant, Illinois

RESOURCES*

American Association of College of Osteopathic Medicine®
(AACOMAS®): http://www.aacom.org.

Association of American Medical Colleges® (AAMC®): www.
aamc.org. The AAMC® represents accredited United States
and Canadian medical schools. At this site, you can also
purchase the book, Medical School Admission Requirements,
which is published annually.

Association of American Medical Colleges® Applicant,
Matriculant, and Enrollment Data: www.aamc.org/data/
facts. Use these data to see how you compare with other
applicants and matriculants.

American Medical College Application Service® (AMCAS®)
Applicant Resources: https://www.aamc.org/students/
applying/. Read the official AMCAS® instructions, course
classification guide, grade conversion guide, and more.

American Medical College Application Service® (AMCAS®):
https://www.aamc.org/students/applying/ amcas. Centralized
application to apply to participating medical schools in the

United States.

American Medical College Application Service® Letter Writer
Application: https://services.aamc.org/ letterwriter. System
through which letter writers can upload letters directly to
AMCAS®.

Free Application for Federal Student Aid (FAFSA®):
http://www.fafsa.ed.gov/.

Medical College Admissions Test®: https://www.aamc.org/
students/applying/mcat Through this portal, you can register
for the MCAT®, find out about current fees, read MCAT®
Essentials, access MCAT® practice tests and more.

Medical School Admissions Requirements®: Published
annually, this must have resource is available in print and
online versions: https://www.aamc.org/students/applying/
requirements/msar/.

National Residency Matching Program® (NRMP®):
www. nrmp.org. The "main" residency match. Site contains
useful information and data about different specialty matches.

Texas Medical and Dental School Application Service®:
http://www.utsystem.edu/tmdsas/. Apply to Texas medical
schools through this application.

*Some websites for these resources change annually.

Made in the USA
Middletown, DE
22 July 2019